MY YOGA JOURNEY

A GUIDED JOURNAL

KASSANDRA REINHARDT
OF YOGA WITH KASSANDRA

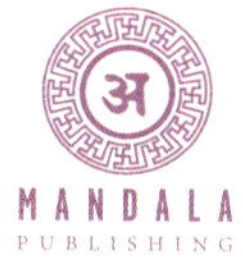

MANDALA
PUBLISHING

MY YOGA JOURNEY: A GUIDED JOURNAL IS YOUR COMPANION TO A DEEPER AND MORE MEANINGFUL YOGA PRACTICE.

It's intended to help you get more out of your time on the mat by taking just two minutes before and after your yoga session to reflect and connect. You can bring this journal with you to your local yoga studio or leave it next to your mat at home for use during your own personal practice.

To use this journal, fill out the date at the top of the page and write down your desired affirmation. An affirmation is a simple, positive statement phrased in the present tense. It should make you feel inspired and focused for your practice. For example: "I love every cell in my body." You can invent your own or use the companion card deck, *I Radiate Joy: Daily Affirmation Cards from Yoga with Kassandra*, for inspiration.

Before you begin your work on the mat, ask yourself what you need from today's practice and use that to set your intention. When thinking of an intention, consider your physical, mental, emotional, and spiritual needs in that moment. Fill out the "Before Yoga" section of the journal while keeping these things in mind. Release judgement and expectation, and write from the heart.

When you're done practicing, fill out the "After Yoga" portion of the journal by noting down which activities you did. You can then summarize your experience using three words and answer the daily prompt. These prompts rotate daily, and there are thirty in total. At the end of each entry, you'll find a bit of extra space to write down anything else that's on your mind.

This journal also includes a Habit Tracker which is a great tool for accountability and motivation. Color in the corresponding date every time you practice yoga and complete your journal entry.

Remember, this process isn't meant to be overwhelming or cumbersome. Keep it short, simple, and to the point. Sometimes the magic is in simplicity and repetition.

After using this journal, my hope is that you will feel deeply connected to your practice and more in tune with yourself. Beginning your practice by setting a clear intention and then reflecting on your experience in the end is an amazing way to cultivate self-awareness and personal growth.

Happy journaling,

Kassandra

HABIT TRACKER

MY YOGA JOURNEY

JAN

FEB

MAR

APR

MAY

JUN

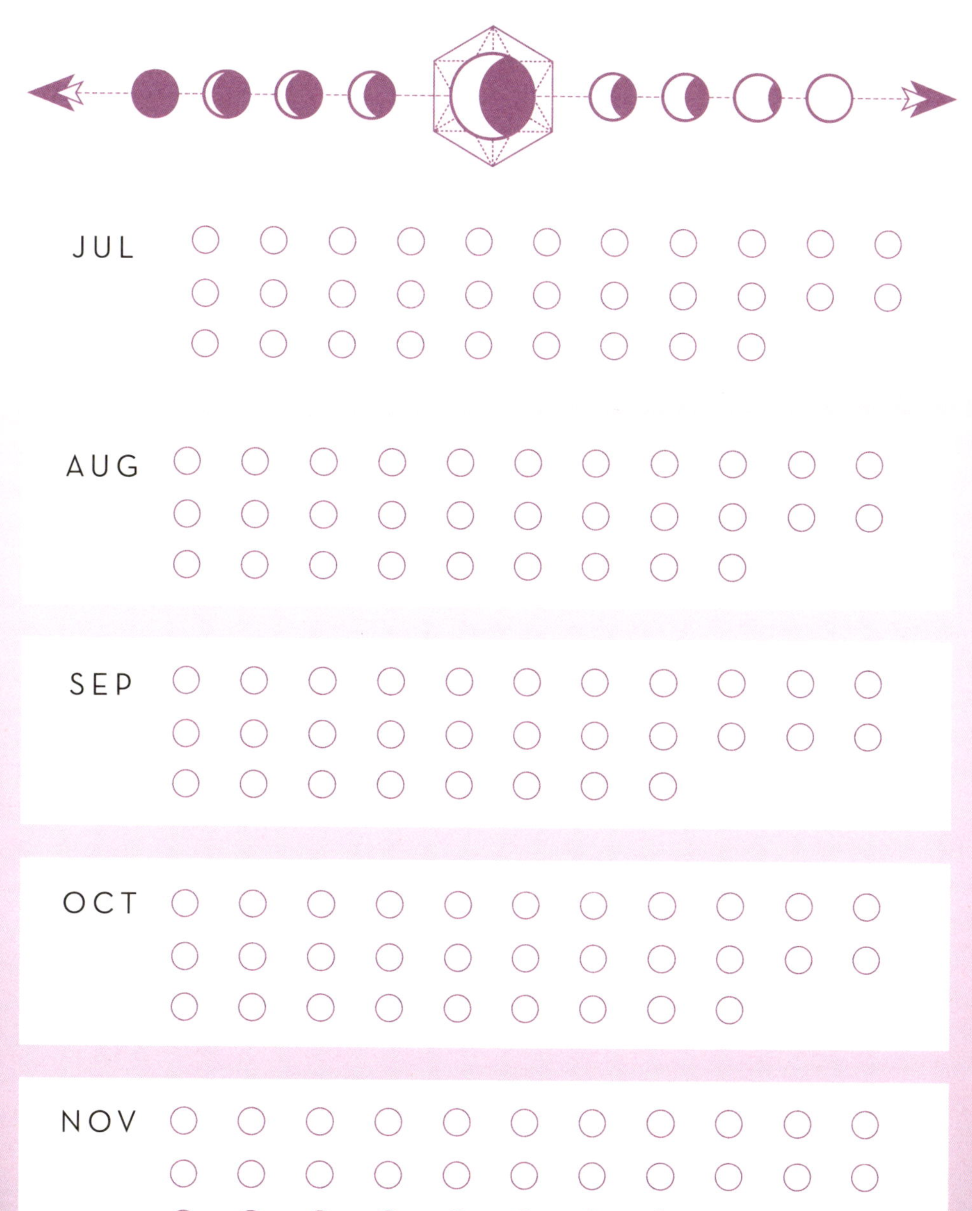
JUL
AUG
SEP
OCT
NOV
DEC

BEFORE YOGA

DATE ___/___/___

AFFIRMATION OF THE DAY:

WHAT DO I NEED FROM TODAY'S PRACTICE?

MY INTENTION IS:

AFTER YOGA

TODAY'S PRACTICE INCLUDED:

- ☐ yoga poses (*asana*)
- ☐ breathwork (*pranayama*)
- ☐ meditation (*dhyana*)
- ☐ chanting mantra
- ☐ other: ______________

3 WORDS THAT CAPTURE HOW MY PRACTICE WENT:

WHAT STOOD OUT MOST ABOUT TODAY'S PRACTICE?

OTHER THOUGHTS:

BEFORE YOGA

DATE ___/___/___

AFFIRMATION OF THE DAY:

WHAT DO I NEED FROM TODAY'S PRACTICE?

MY INTENTION IS:

AFTER YOGA

TODAY'S PRACTICE INCLUDED:

- ☐ yoga poses (*asana*)
- ☐ breathwork (*pranayama*)
- ☐ meditation (*dhyana*)
- ☐ chanting mantra
- ☐ other: ___

3 WORDS THAT CAPTURE HOW MY PRACTICE WENT:

WHAT AM I MOST PROUD OF?

OTHER THOUGHTS:

BEFORE YOGA

DATE ___/___/___

AFFIRMATION OF THE DAY:

WHAT DO I NEED FROM TODAY'S PRACTICE?

MY INTENTION IS:

AFTER YOGA

TODAY'S PRACTICE INCLUDED:

- ☐ yoga poses (*asana*)
- ☐ breathwork (*pranayama*)
- ☐ meditation (*dhyana*)
- ☐ chanting mantra
- ☐ other: ________

3 WORDS THAT CAPTURE HOW MY PRACTICE WENT:

WHAT WAS THE HARDEST PART OF TODAY'S PRACTICE?

OTHER THOUGHTS:

BEFORE YOGA

DATE ___/___/___

AFFIRMATION OF THE DAY:

WHAT DO I NEED FROM TODAY'S PRACTICE?

MY INTENTION IS:

AFTER YOGA

TODAY'S PRACTICE INCLUDED:

- ☐ yoga poses (*asana*)
- ☐ breathwork (*pranayama*)
- ☐ meditation (*dhyana*)
- ☐ chanting mantra
- ☐ other: ________

3 WORDS THAT CAPTURE HOW MY PRACTICE WENT:

WHAT DID I LEARN ABOUT MYSELF?

OTHER THOUGHTS:

BEFORE YOGA

DATE ___/___/___

AFFIRMATION OF THE DAY:

WHAT DO I NEED FROM TODAY'S PRACTICE?

MY INTENTION IS:

AFTER YOGA

TODAY'S PRACTICE INCLUDED:

- ☐ yoga poses (*asana*)
- ☐ breathwork (*pranayama*)
- ☐ meditation (*dhyana*)
- ☐ chanting mantra
- ☐ other: ___

3 WORDS THAT CAPTURE HOW MY PRACTICE WENT:

HOW CAN I TAKE MY YOGA OFF THE MAT AND INTO THE WORLD?

OTHER THOUGHTS:

BEFORE YOGA

DATE ___/___/___

AFFIRMATION OF THE DAY:

WHAT DO I NEED FROM TODAY'S PRACTICE?

MY INTENTION IS:

AFTER YOGA

TODAY'S PRACTICE INCLUDED:

- ☐ yoga poses (*asana*)
- ☐ breathwork (*pranayama*)
- ☐ meditation (*dhyana*)
- ☐ chanting mantra
- ☐ other: ___________

3 WORDS THAT CAPTURE HOW MY PRACTICE WENT:

WHAT DOES YOGA MEAN TO ME?

OTHER THOUGHTS:

BEFORE YOGA

DATE ___/___/___

AFFIRMATION OF THE DAY:

WHAT DO I NEED FROM TODAY'S PRACTICE?

MY INTENTION IS:

AFTER YOGA

TODAY'S PRACTICE INCLUDED:

- ☐ yoga poses (*asana*)
- ☐ breathwork (*pranayama*)
- ☐ meditation (*dhyana*)
- ☐ chanting mantra
- ☐ other: __________

3 WORDS THAT CAPTURE HOW MY PRACTICE WENT:

HOW CONNECTED WAS I TO MY BREATH?

OTHER THOUGHTS:

BEFORE YOGA

DATE ___/___/___

AFFIRMATION OF THE DAY:

WHAT DO I NEED FROM TODAY'S PRACTICE?

MY INTENTION IS:

AFTER YOGA

TODAY'S PRACTICE INCLUDED:

- [ ] yoga poses (*asana*)
- [ ] breathwork (*pranayama*)
- [ ] meditation (*dhyana*)
- [ ] chanting mantra
- [ ] other: __________

3 WORDS THAT CAPTURE HOW MY PRACTICE WENT:

HOW DO I FEEL ABOUT MY BODY RIGHT NOW?

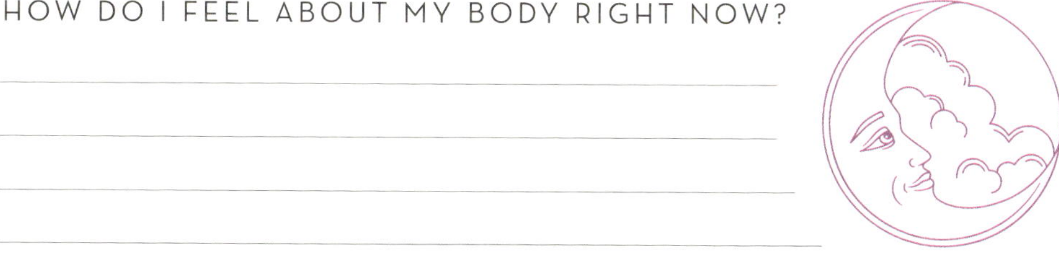

OTHER THOUGHTS:

BEFORE YOGA

DATE ___/___/___

AFFIRMATION OF THE DAY:

WHAT DO I NEED FROM TODAY'S PRACTICE?

MY INTENTION IS:

AFTER YOGA

TODAY'S PRACTICE INCLUDED:

- ☐ yoga poses (*asana*)
- ☐ breathwork (*pranayama*)
- ☐ meditation (*dhyana*)
- ☐ chanting mantra
- ☐ other: ___

3 WORDS THAT CAPTURE HOW MY PRACTICE WENT:

DID I HONOR MY INTENTION DURING PRACTICE?

OTHER THOUGHTS:

BEFORE YOGA

DATE ___/___/___

AFFIRMATION OF THE DAY:

WHAT DO I NEED FROM TODAY'S PRACTICE?

MY INTENTION IS:

AFTER YOGA

TODAY'S PRACTICE INCLUDED:

- ☐ yoga poses (*asana*)
- ☐ breathwork (*pranayama*)
- ☐ meditation (*dhyana*)
- ☐ chanting mantra
- ☐ other: ________

3 WORDS THAT CAPTURE HOW MY PRACTICE WENT:

WHAT WAS THE MAIN EMOTION FELT DURING PRACTICE?

OTHER THOUGHTS:

BEFORE YOGA

DATE ___/___/___

AFFIRMATION OF THE DAY:

WHAT DO I NEED FROM TODAY'S PRACTICE?

MY INTENTION IS:

AFTER YOGA

TODAY'S PRACTICE INCLUDED:

- ☐ yoga poses (*asana*)
- ☐ breathwork (*pranayama*)
- ☐ meditation (*dhyana*)
- ☐ chanting mantra
- ☐ other: ______

3 WORDS THAT CAPTURE HOW MY PRACTICE WENT:

HOW DO I REACT WHEN FACED WITH A CHALLENGING POSE OR PRACTICE?

OTHER THOUGHTS:

BEFORE YOGA

DATE ___/___/___

AFFIRMATION OF THE DAY:

WHAT DO I NEED FROM TODAY'S PRACTICE?

MY INTENTION IS:

AFTER YOGA

TODAY'S PRACTICE INCLUDED:

- ☐ yoga poses (*asana*)
- ☐ breathwork (*pranayama*)
- ☐ meditation (*dhyana*)
- ☐ chanting mantra
- ☐ other: __________

3 WORDS THAT CAPTURE HOW MY PRACTICE WENT:

HOW ARE EVENTS IN MY LIFE AFFECTING MY PRACTICE?

OTHER THOUGHTS:

BEFORE YOGA

DATE ___/___/___

AFFIRMATION OF THE DAY:

WHAT DO I NEED FROM TODAY'S PRACTICE?

MY INTENTION IS:

AFTER YOGA

TODAY'S PRACTICE INCLUDED:

- ☐ yoga poses (*asana*)
- ☐ breathwork (*pranayama*)
- ☐ meditation (*dhyana*)
- ☐ chanting mantra
- ☐ other: ___________

3 WORDS THAT CAPTURE HOW MY PRACTICE WENT:

HOW DOES MY PRACTICE AFFECT MY DAY-TO-DAY LIFE?

OTHER THOUGHTS:

BEFORE YOGA

DATE ___/___/___

AFFIRMATION OF THE DAY:

WHAT DO I NEED FROM TODAY'S PRACTICE?

MY INTENTION IS:

AFTER YOGA

TODAY'S PRACTICE INCLUDED:

- ☐ yoga poses (*asana*)
- ☐ breathwork (*pranayama*)
- ☐ meditation (*dhyana*)
- ☐ chanting mantra
- ☐ other: __________

3 WORDS THAT CAPTURE HOW MY PRACTICE WENT:

HOW CAN I USE THIS PRACTICE FOR SPIRITUAL GROWTH?

OTHER THOUGHTS:

BEFORE YOGA

DATE ___/___/___

AFFIRMATION OF THE DAY:

WHAT DO I NEED FROM TODAY'S PRACTICE?

MY INTENTION IS:

AFTER YOGA

TODAY'S PRACTICE INCLUDED:

- ☐ yoga poses (*asana*)
- ☐ breathwork (*pranayama*)
- ☐ meditation (*dhyana*)
- ☐ chanting mantra
- ☐ other: ______________

3 WORDS THAT CAPTURE HOW MY PRACTICE WENT:

HOW EASY OR DIFFICULT WAS IT FOR ME TO STAY FOCUSED?

OTHER THOUGHTS:

BEFORE YOGA

DATE ___/___/___

AFFIRMATION OF THE DAY:

WHAT DO I NEED FROM TODAY'S PRACTICE?

MY INTENTION IS:

AFTER YOGA

TODAY'S PRACTICE INCLUDED:

- ☐ yoga poses (*asana*)
- ☐ breathwork (*pranayama*)
- ☐ meditation (*dhyana*)
- ☐ chanting mantra
- ☐ other: ___________

3 WORDS THAT CAPTURE HOW MY PRACTICE WENT:

WHAT HELPS ME STAY IN THE PRESENT MOMENT?

OTHER THOUGHTS:

BEFORE YOGA

DATE ___/___/___

AFFIRMATION OF THE DAY:

WHAT DO I NEED FROM TODAY'S PRACTICE?

MY INTENTION IS:

AFTER YOGA

TODAY'S PRACTICE INCLUDED:

- ☐ yoga poses (*asana*)
- ☐ breathwork (*pranayama*)
- ☐ meditation (*dhyana*)
- ☐ chanting mantra
- ☐ other: ____________

3 WORDS THAT CAPTURE HOW MY PRACTICE WENT:

WHICH TEACHERS DO I FIND MOST INSPIRING AND WHY?

OTHER THOUGHTS:

BEFORE YOGA

DATE ___/___/___

AFFIRMATION OF THE DAY:

WHAT DO I NEED FROM TODAY'S PRACTICE?

MY INTENTION IS:

AFTER YOGA

TODAY'S PRACTICE INCLUDED:

- ☐ yoga poses (*asana*)
- ☐ breathwork (*pranayama*)
- ☐ meditation (*dhyana*)
- ☐ chanting mantra
- ☐ other: ____________

3 WORDS THAT CAPTURE HOW MY PRACTICE WENT:

IF I COULD CHANGE ANYTHING FROM TODAY'S PRACTICE, WHAT WOULD IT BE?

OTHER THOUGHTS:

BEFORE YOGA

DATE ___/___/___

AFFIRMATION OF THE DAY:

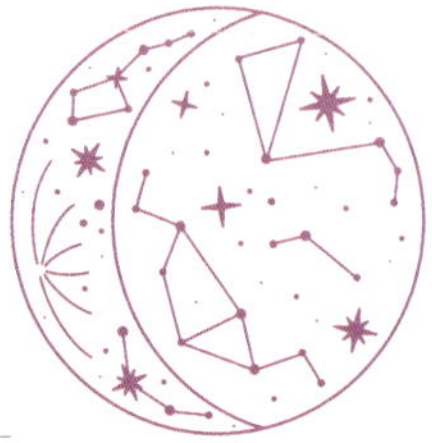

WHAT DO I NEED FROM TODAY'S PRACTICE?

MY INTENTION IS:

AFTER YOGA

TODAY'S PRACTICE INCLUDED:

- ☐ yoga poses (*asana*)
- ☐ breathwork (*pranayama*)
- ☐ meditation (*dhyana*)
- ☐ chanting mantra
- ☐ other: ___________

3 WORDS THAT CAPTURE HOW MY PRACTICE WENT:

DO I TEND TO PUSH TOO HARD OR HOLD BACK?

OTHER THOUGHTS:

BEFORE YOGA

DATE ___/___/___

AFFIRMATION OF THE DAY:

WHAT DO I NEED FROM TODAY'S PRACTICE?

MY INTENTION IS:

AFTER YOGA

TODAY'S PRACTICE INCLUDED:

- ☐ yoga poses (*asana*)
- ☐ breathwork (*pranayama*)
- ☐ meditation (*dhyana*)
- ☐ chanting mantra
- ☐ other: ___________

3 WORDS THAT CAPTURE HOW MY PRACTICE WENT:

WHAT MOTIVATES ME TO KEEP PRACTICING EVERY DAY?

OTHER THOUGHTS:

BEFORE YOGA

DATE ___/___/___

AFFIRMATION OF THE DAY:

WHAT DO I NEED FROM TODAY'S PRACTICE?

MY INTENTION IS:

AFTER YOGA

TODAY'S PRACTICE INCLUDED:

- ☐ yoga poses (*asana*)
- ☐ breathwork (*pranayama*)
- ☐ meditation (*dhyana*)
- ☐ chanting mantra
- ☐ other: ________

3 WORDS THAT CAPTURE HOW MY PRACTICE WENT:

HOW HAS MY RELATIONSHIP WITH YOGA CHANGED WITH TIME?

OTHER THOUGHTS:

BEFORE YOGA

DATE ___/___/___

AFFIRMATION OF THE DAY:

WHAT DO I NEED FROM TODAY'S PRACTICE?

MY INTENTION IS:

AFTER YOGA

TODAY'S PRACTICE INCLUDED:

- ☐ yoga poses (*asana*)
- ☐ breathwork (*pranayama*)
- ☐ meditation (*dhyana*)
- ☐ chanting mantra
- ☐ other: ___

3 WORDS THAT CAPTURE HOW MY PRACTICE WENT:

WHAT DO I NEED MORE OF IN MY PRACTICE?

OTHER THOUGHTS:

BEFORE YOGA

DATE ___/___/___

AFFIRMATION OF THE DAY:

WHAT DO I NEED FROM TODAY'S PRACTICE?

MY INTENTION IS:

AFTER YOGA

TODAY'S PRACTICE INCLUDED:

- ☐ yoga poses (*asana*)
- ☐ breathwork (*pranayama*)
- ☐ meditation (*dhyana*)
- ☐ chanting mantra
- ☐ other: __________

3 WORDS THAT CAPTURE HOW MY PRACTICE WENT:

WHAT DO I WANT TO WORK ON NEXT TIME?

OTHER THOUGHTS:

BEFORE YOGA

DATE ___/___/___

AFFIRMATION OF THE DAY:

____

WHAT DO I NEED FROM TODAY'S PRACTICE?

____

____

____

MY INTENTION IS:

____

____

AFTER YOGA

TODAY'S PRACTICE INCLUDED:

- ☐ yoga poses (*asana*)
- ☐ breathwork (*pranayama*)
- ☐ meditation (*dhyana*)
- ☐ chanting mantra
- ☐ other: ______________

3 WORDS THAT CAPTURE HOW MY PRACTICE WENT:

____

____

____

AM I NEGLECTING AN IMPORTANT ASPECT OF MY YOGA PRACTICE?

____

____

____

OTHER THOUGHTS:

____

____

____

BEFORE YOGA

DATE ___/___/___

AFFIRMATION OF THE DAY:

WHAT DO I NEED FROM TODAY'S PRACTICE?

MY INTENTION IS:

AFTER YOGA

TODAY'S PRACTICE INCLUDED:

- ☐ yoga poses (*asana*)
- ☐ breathwork (*pranayama*)
- ☐ meditation (*dhyana*)
- ☐ chanting mantra
- ☐ other: ___

3 WORDS THAT CAPTURE HOW MY PRACTICE WENT:

DOES MY INTERNAL DIALOGUE TEND TO BE POSITIVE OR NEGATIVE?

OTHER THOUGHTS:

BEFORE YOGA

DATE ___/___/___

AFFIRMATION OF THE DAY:

WHAT DO I NEED FROM TODAY'S PRACTICE?

MY INTENTION IS:

AFTER YOGA

TODAY'S PRACTICE INCLUDED:

- ☐ yoga poses (*asana*)
- ☐ breathwork (*pranayama*)
- ☐ meditation (*dhyana*)
- ☐ chanting mantra
- ☐ other: ______________

3 WORDS THAT CAPTURE HOW MY PRACTICE WENT:

WHAT AM I MOST GRATEFUL FOR RIGHT NOW?

OTHER THOUGHTS:

BEFORE YOGA

DATE ___/___/___

AFFIRMATION OF THE DAY:

WHAT DO I NEED FROM TODAY'S PRACTICE?

MY INTENTION IS:

AFTER YOGA

TODAY'S PRACTICE INCLUDED:

- ☐ yoga poses (*asana*)
- ☐ breathwork (*pranayama*)
- ☐ meditation (*dhyana*)
- ☐ chanting mantra
- ☐ other: ___________

3 WORDS THAT CAPTURE HOW MY PRACTICE WENT:

WHAT IS SOMETHING I NEED TO STUDY DEEPER?

OTHER THOUGHTS:

BEFORE YOGA

DATE ___/___/___

AFFIRMATION OF THE DAY:

WHAT DO I NEED FROM TODAY'S PRACTICE?

MY INTENTION IS:

AFTER YOGA

TODAY'S PRACTICE INCLUDED:

- ☐ yoga poses (*asana*)
- ☐ breathwork (*pranayama*)
- ☐ meditation (*dhyana*)
- ☐ chanting mantra
- ☐ other: ___________

3 WORDS THAT CAPTURE HOW MY PRACTICE WENT:

HOW DOES YOGA AFFECT MY EMOTIONAL HEALTH?

OTHER THOUGHTS:

BEFORE YOGA

DATE ___/___/___

AFFIRMATION OF THE DAY:

WHAT DO I NEED FROM TODAY'S PRACTICE?

MY INTENTION IS:

AFTER YOGA

TODAY'S PRACTICE INCLUDED:

- ☐ yoga poses (*asana*)
- ☐ breathwork (*pranayama*)
- ☐ meditation (*dhyana*)
- ☐ chanting mantra
- ☐ other: ___

3 WORDS THAT CAPTURE HOW MY PRACTICE WENT:

HOW DID THIS PRACTICE AFFECT MY ENERGY LEVELS?

OTHER THOUGHTS:

BEFORE YOGA

DATE ___/___/___

AFFIRMATION OF THE DAY:

WHAT DO I NEED FROM TODAY'S PRACTICE?

MY INTENTION IS:

AFTER YOGA

TODAY'S PRACTICE INCLUDED:

- ☐ yoga poses (*asana*)
- ☐ breathwork (*pranayama*)
- ☐ meditation (*dhyana*)
- ☐ chanting mantra
- ☐ other: ___

3 WORDS THAT CAPTURE HOW MY PRACTICE WENT:

HOW DOES YOGA CONNECT ME WITH MY PURPOSE?

OTHER THOUGHTS:

BEFORE YOGA

DATE ___/___/___

AFFIRMATION OF THE DAY:

WHAT DO I NEED FROM TODAY'S PRACTICE?

MY INTENTION IS:

AFTER YOGA

TODAY'S PRACTICE INCLUDED:

- ☐ yoga poses (*asana*)
- ☐ breathwork (*pranayama*)
- ☐ meditation (*dhyana*)
- ☐ chanting mantra
- ☐ other: ______

3 WORDS THAT CAPTURE HOW MY PRACTICE WENT:

WHAT STOOD OUT MOST ABOUT TODAY'S PRACTICE?

OTHER THOUGHTS:

BEFORE YOGA

DATE ___/___/___

AFFIRMATION OF THE DAY:

WHAT DO I NEED FROM TODAY'S PRACTICE?

MY INTENTION IS:

AFTER YOGA

TODAY'S PRACTICE INCLUDED:

- ☐ yoga poses (*asana*)
- ☐ breathwork (*pranayama*)
- ☐ meditation (*dhyana*)
- ☐ chanting mantra
- ☐ other: __________

3 WORDS THAT CAPTURE HOW MY PRACTICE WENT:

WHAT AM I MOST PROUD OF?

OTHER THOUGHTS:

BEFORE YOGA

DATE ___/___/___

AFFIRMATION OF THE DAY:

WHAT DO I NEED FROM TODAY'S PRACTICE?

MY INTENTION IS:

AFTER YOGA

TODAY'S PRACTICE INCLUDED:

- ☐ yoga poses (*asana*)
- ☐ breathwork (*pranayama*)
- ☐ meditation (*dhyana*)
- ☐ chanting mantra
- ☐ other: __________

3 WORDS THAT CAPTURE HOW MY PRACTICE WENT:

WHAT WAS THE HARDEST PART OF TODAY'S PRACTICE?

OTHER THOUGHTS:

BEFORE YOGA

DATE ___/___/___

AFFIRMATION OF THE DAY:

WHAT DO I NEED FROM TODAY'S PRACTICE?

MY INTENTION IS:

AFTER YOGA

TODAY'S PRACTICE INCLUDED:

- ☐ yoga poses (*asana*)
- ☐ breathwork (*pranayama*)
- ☐ meditation (*dhyana*)
- ☐ chanting mantra
- ☐ other: ______

3 WORDS THAT CAPTURE HOW MY PRACTICE WENT:

WHAT DID I LEARN ABOUT MYSELF?

OTHER THOUGHTS:

BEFORE YOGA

DATE ___/___/___

AFFIRMATION OF THE DAY:

WHAT DO I NEED FROM TODAY'S PRACTICE?

MY INTENTION IS:

AFTER YOGA

TODAY'S PRACTICE INCLUDED:

- ☐ yoga poses (*asana*)
- ☐ breathwork (*pranayama*)
- ☐ meditation (*dhyana*)
- ☐ chanting mantra
- ☐ other: ___

3 WORDS THAT CAPTURE HOW MY PRACTICE WENT:

HOW CAN I TAKE MY YOGA OFF THE MAT AND INTO THE WORLD?

OTHER THOUGHTS:

BEFORE YOGA

DATE ___/___/___

AFFIRMATION OF THE DAY:

WHAT DO I NEED FROM TODAY'S PRACTICE?

MY INTENTION IS:

AFTER YOGA

TODAY'S PRACTICE INCLUDED:

- ☐ yoga poses (*asana*)
- ☐ breathwork (*pranayama*)
- ☐ meditation (*dhyana*)
- ☐ chanting mantra
- ☐ other: ________

3 WORDS THAT CAPTURE HOW MY PRACTICE WENT:

WHAT DOES YOGA MEAN TO ME?

OTHER THOUGHTS:

BEFORE YOGA

DATE ___/___/___

AFFIRMATION OF THE DAY:

WHAT DO I NEED FROM TODAY'S PRACTICE?

MY INTENTION IS:

AFTER YOGA

TODAY'S PRACTICE INCLUDED:

- ☐ yoga poses (*asana*)
- ☐ breathwork (*pranayama*)
- ☐ meditation (*dhyana*)
- ☐ chanting mantra
- ☐ other: __________

3 WORDS THAT CAPTURE HOW MY PRACTICE WENT:

HOW CONNECTED WAS I TO MY BREATH?

OTHER THOUGHTS:

BEFORE YOGA

DATE ___/___/___

AFFIRMATION OF THE DAY:

WHAT DO I NEED FROM TODAY'S PRACTICE?

MY INTENTION IS:

AFTER YOGA

TODAY'S PRACTICE INCLUDED:

- ☐ yoga poses (*asana*)
- ☐ breathwork (*pranayama*)
- ☐ meditation (*dhyana*)
- ☐ chanting mantra
- ☐ other: ____________

3 WORDS THAT CAPTURE HOW MY PRACTICE WENT:

HOW DO I FEEL ABOUT MY BODY RIGHT NOW?

OTHER THOUGHTS:

BEFORE YOGA

DATE ___/___/___

AFFIRMATION OF THE DAY:

WHAT DO I NEED FROM TODAY'S PRACTICE?

MY INTENTION IS:

AFTER YOGA

TODAY'S PRACTICE INCLUDED:

- ☐ yoga poses (*asana*)
- ☐ breathwork (*pranayama*)
- ☐ meditation (*dhyana*)
- ☐ chanting mantra
- ☐ other: __________

3 WORDS THAT CAPTURE HOW MY PRACTICE WENT:

DID I HONOR MY INTENTION DURING PRACTICE?

OTHER THOUGHTS:

BEFORE YOGA

DATE ___/___/___

AFFIRMATION OF THE DAY:

WHAT DO I NEED FROM TODAY'S PRACTICE?

MY INTENTION IS:

AFTER YOGA

TODAY'S PRACTICE INCLUDED:

- ☐ yoga poses (*asana*)
- ☐ breathwork (*pranayama*)
- ☐ meditation (*dhyana*)
- ☐ chanting mantra
- ☐ other: ___________

3 WORDS THAT CAPTURE HOW MY PRACTICE WENT:

WHAT WAS THE MAIN EMOTION FELT DURING PRACTICE?

OTHER THOUGHTS:

BEFORE YOGA

DATE ___/___/___

AFFIRMATION OF THE DAY:

WHAT DO I NEED FROM TODAY'S PRACTICE?

MY INTENTION IS:

AFTER YOGA

TODAY'S PRACTICE INCLUDED:

- ☐ yoga poses (*asana*)
- ☐ breathwork (*pranayama*)
- ☐ meditation (*dhyana*)
- ☐ chanting mantra
- ☐ other: ___

3 WORDS THAT CAPTURE HOW MY PRACTICE WENT:

HOW DO I REACT WHEN FACED WITH A CHALLENGING POSE OR PRACTICE?

OTHER THOUGHTS:

BEFORE YOGA

DATE ___/___/___

AFFIRMATION OF THE DAY:

WHAT DO I NEED FROM TODAY'S PRACTICE?

MY INTENTION IS:

AFTER YOGA

TODAY'S PRACTICE INCLUDED:

- ☐ yoga poses (*asana*)
- ☐ breathwork (*pranayama*)
- ☐ meditation (*dhyana*)
- ☐ chanting mantra
- ☐ other: ___

3 WORDS THAT CAPTURE HOW MY PRACTICE WENT:

HOW ARE EVENTS IN MY LIFE AFFECTING MY PRACTICE?

OTHER THOUGHTS:

BEFORE YOGA

DATE ___/___/___

AFFIRMATION OF THE DAY:

WHAT DO I NEED FROM TODAY'S PRACTICE?

MY INTENTION IS:

AFTER YOGA

TODAY'S PRACTICE INCLUDED:

- ☐ yoga poses (*asana*)
- ☐ breathwork (*pranayama*)
- ☐ meditation (*dhyana*)
- ☐ chanting mantra
- ☐ other: ___

3 WORDS THAT CAPTURE HOW MY PRACTICE WENT:

HOW DOES MY PRACTICE AFFECT MY DAY-TO-DAY LIFE?

OTHER THOUGHTS:

BEFORE YOGA

DATE ___/___/___

AFFIRMATION OF THE DAY:

WHAT DO I NEED FROM TODAY'S PRACTICE?

MY INTENTION IS:

AFTER YOGA

TODAY'S PRACTICE INCLUDED:

- ☐ yoga poses (*asana*)
- ☐ breathwork (*pranayama*)
- ☐ meditation (*dhyana*)
- ☐ chanting mantra
- ☐ other: ____________

3 WORDS THAT CAPTURE HOW MY PRACTICE WENT:

HOW CAN I USE THIS PRACTICE FOR SPIRITUAL GROWTH?

OTHER THOUGHTS:

BEFORE YOGA

DATE ___/___/___

AFFIRMATION OF THE DAY:

WHAT DO I NEED FROM TODAY'S PRACTICE?

MY INTENTION IS:

AFTER YOGA

TODAY'S PRACTICE INCLUDED:

- ☐ yoga poses (*asana*)
- ☐ breathwork (*pranayama*)
- ☐ meditation (*dhyana*)
- ☐ chanting mantra
- ☐ other: ___

3 WORDS THAT CAPTURE HOW MY PRACTICE WENT:

HOW EASY OR DIFFICULT WAS IT FOR ME TO STAY FOCUSED?

OTHER THOUGHTS:

BEFORE YOGA

DATE ___/___/___

AFFIRMATION OF THE DAY:

WHAT DO I NEED FROM TODAY'S PRACTICE?

MY INTENTION IS:

AFTER YOGA

TODAY'S PRACTICE INCLUDED:

- ☐ yoga poses (*asana*)
- ☐ breathwork (*pranayama*)
- ☐ meditation (*dhyana*)
- ☐ chanting mantra
- ☐ other: __________

3 WORDS THAT CAPTURE HOW MY PRACTICE WENT:

WHAT HELPS ME STAY IN THE PRESENT MOMENT?

OTHER THOUGHTS:

BEFORE YOGA

DATE ___/___/___

AFFIRMATION OF THE DAY:

WHAT DO I NEED FROM TODAY'S PRACTICE?

MY INTENTION IS:

AFTER YOGA

TODAY'S PRACTICE INCLUDED:

- ☐ yoga poses (*asana*)
- ☐ breathwork (*pranayama*)
- ☐ meditation (*dhyana*)
- ☐ chanting mantra
- ☐ other: __________

3 WORDS THAT CAPTURE HOW MY PRACTICE WENT:

WHICH TEACHERS DO I FIND MOST INSPIRING AND WHY?

OTHER THOUGHTS:

BEFORE YOGA

DATE ___/___/___

AFFIRMATION OF THE DAY:

WHAT DO I NEED FROM TODAY'S PRACTICE?

MY INTENTION IS:

AFTER YOGA

TODAY'S PRACTICE INCLUDED:

- ☐ yoga poses (*asana*)
- ☐ breathwork (*pranayama*)
- ☐ meditation (*dhyana*)
- ☐ chanting mantra
- ☐ other: ______________

3 WORDS THAT CAPTURE HOW MY PRACTICE WENT:

IF I COULD CHANGE ANYTHING FROM TODAY'S PRACTICE, WHAT WOULD IT BE?

OTHER THOUGHTS:

BEFORE YOGA

DATE ___/___/___

AFFIRMATION OF THE DAY:

WHAT DO I NEED FROM TODAY'S PRACTICE?

MY INTENTION IS:

AFTER YOGA

TODAY'S PRACTICE INCLUDED:

- ☐ yoga poses (*asana*)
- ☐ breathwork (*pranayama*)
- ☐ meditation (*dhyana*)
- ☐ chanting mantra
- ☐ other: ________

3 WORDS THAT CAPTURE HOW MY PRACTICE WENT:

DO I TEND TO PUSH TOO HARD OR HOLD BACK?

OTHER THOUGHTS:

BEFORE YOGA

DATE ___/___/___

AFFIRMATION OF THE DAY:

WHAT DO I NEED FROM TODAY'S PRACTICE?

MY INTENTION IS:

AFTER YOGA

TODAY'S PRACTICE INCLUDED:

- ☐ yoga poses (*asana*)
- ☐ breathwork (*pranayama*)
- ☐ meditation (*dhyana*)
- ☐ chanting mantra
- ☐ other: ________

3 WORDS THAT CAPTURE HOW MY PRACTICE WENT:

WHAT MOTIVATES ME TO KEEP PRACTICING EVERY DAY?

OTHER THOUGHTS:

BEFORE YOGA

DATE ___/___/___

AFFIRMATION OF THE DAY:

WHAT DO I NEED FROM TODAY'S PRACTICE?

MY INTENTION IS:

AFTER YOGA

TODAY'S PRACTICE INCLUDED:

- ☐ yoga poses (*asana*)
- ☐ breathwork (*pranayama*)
- ☐ meditation (*dhyana*)
- ☐ chanting mantra
- ☐ other: ____________

3 WORDS THAT CAPTURE HOW MY PRACTICE WENT:

HOW HAS MY RELATIONSHIP WITH YOGA CHANGED WITH TIME?

OTHER THOUGHTS:

BEFORE YOGA

DATE ___/___/___

AFFIRMATION OF THE DAY:

WHAT DO I NEED FROM TODAY'S PRACTICE?

MY INTENTION IS:

AFTER YOGA

TODAY'S PRACTICE INCLUDED:

- ☐ yoga poses (*asana*)
- ☐ breathwork (*pranayama*)
- ☐ meditation (*dhyana*)
- ☐ chanting mantra
- ☐ other: ______________

3 WORDS THAT CAPTURE HOW MY PRACTICE WENT:

WHAT DO I NEED MORE OF IN MY PRACTICE?

OTHER THOUGHTS:

BEFORE YOGA

DATE ___/___/___

AFFIRMATION OF THE DAY:

WHAT DO I NEED FROM TODAY'S PRACTICE?

MY INTENTION IS:

AFTER YOGA

TODAY'S PRACTICE INCLUDED:

- ☐ yoga poses (*asana*)
- ☐ breathwork (*pranayama*)
- ☐ meditation (*dhyana*)
- ☐ chanting mantra
- ☐ other: __________

3 WORDS THAT CAPTURE HOW MY PRACTICE WENT:

WHAT DO I WANT TO WORK ON NEXT TIME?

OTHER THOUGHTS:

BEFORE YOGA

DATE ___/___/___

AFFIRMATION OF THE DAY:

WHAT DO I NEED FROM TODAY'S PRACTICE?

MY INTENTION IS:

AFTER YOGA

TODAY'S PRACTICE INCLUDED:

- ☐ yoga poses (*asana*)
- ☐ breathwork (*pranayama*)
- ☐ meditation (*dhyana*)
- ☐ chanting mantra
- ☐ other: ___

3 WORDS THAT CAPTURE HOW MY PRACTICE WENT:

AM I NEGLECTING AN IMPORTANT ASPECT OF MY YOGA PRACTICE?

OTHER THOUGHTS:

BEFORE YOGA

DATE ___/___/___

AFFIRMATION OF THE DAY:

WHAT DO I NEED FROM TODAY'S PRACTICE?

MY INTENTION IS:

AFTER YOGA

TODAY'S PRACTICE INCLUDED:

- ☐ yoga poses (*asana*)
- ☐ breathwork (*pranayama*)
- ☐ meditation (*dhyana*)
- ☐ chanting mantra
- ☐ other: ___

3 WORDS THAT CAPTURE HOW MY PRACTICE WENT:

DOES MY INTERNAL DIALOGUE TEND TO BE POSITIVE OR NEGATIVE?

OTHER THOUGHTS:

BEFORE YOGA

DATE ___/___/___

AFFIRMATION OF THE DAY:

WHAT DO I NEED FROM TODAY'S PRACTICE?

MY INTENTION IS:

AFTER YOGA

TODAY'S PRACTICE INCLUDED:

- ☐ yoga poses (*asana*)
- ☐ breathwork (*pranayama*)
- ☐ meditation (*dhyana*)
- ☐ chanting mantra
- ☐ other: ____________

3 WORDS THAT CAPTURE HOW MY PRACTICE WENT:

WHAT AM I MOST GRATEFUL FOR RIGHT NOW?

OTHER THOUGHTS:

BEFORE YOGA

DATE ___/___/___

AFFIRMATION OF THE DAY:

WHAT DO I NEED FROM TODAY'S PRACTICE?

MY INTENTION IS:

AFTER YOGA

TODAY'S PRACTICE INCLUDED:

- ☐ yoga poses (*asana*)
- ☐ breathwork (*pranayama*)
- ☐ meditation (*dhyana*)
- ☐ chanting mantra
- ☐ other: __________

3 WORDS THAT CAPTURE HOW MY PRACTICE WENT:

WHAT IS SOMETHING I NEED TO STUDY DEEPER?

OTHER THOUGHTS:

BEFORE YOGA

DATE ___/___/___

AFFIRMATION OF THE DAY:

WHAT DO I NEED FROM TODAY'S PRACTICE?

MY INTENTION IS:

AFTER YOGA

TODAY'S PRACTICE INCLUDED:

- ☐ yoga poses (*asana*)
- ☐ breathwork (*pranayama*)
- ☐ meditation (*dhyana*)
- ☐ chanting mantra
- ☐ other: ____________

3 WORDS THAT CAPTURE HOW MY PRACTICE WENT:

HOW DOES YOGA AFFECT MY EMOTIONAL HEALTH?

OTHER THOUGHTS:

BEFORE YOGA

DATE ___/___/___

AFFIRMATION OF THE DAY:

WHAT DO I NEED FROM TODAY'S PRACTICE?

MY INTENTION IS:

AFTER YOGA

TODAY'S PRACTICE INCLUDED:

- ☐ yoga poses (*asana*)
- ☐ breathwork (*pranayama*)
- ☐ meditation (*dhyana*)
- ☐ chanting mantra
- ☐ other: ______

3 WORDS THAT CAPTURE HOW MY PRACTICE WENT:

HOW DID THIS PRACTICE AFFECT MY ENERGY LEVELS?

OTHER THOUGHTS:

BEFORE YOGA

DATE ___/___/___

AFFIRMATION OF THE DAY:

WHAT DO I NEED FROM TODAY'S PRACTICE?

MY INTENTION IS:

AFTER YOGA

TODAY'S PRACTICE INCLUDED:

- ☐ yoga poses (*asana*)
- ☐ breathwork (*pranayama*)
- ☐ meditation (*dhyana*)
- ☐ chanting mantra
- ☐ other: ____________

3 WORDS THAT CAPTURE HOW MY PRACTICE WENT:

HOW DOES YOGA CONNECT ME WITH MY PURPOSE?

OTHER THOUGHTS:

BEFORE YOGA

DATE ___/___/___

AFFIRMATION OF THE DAY:

WHAT DO I NEED FROM TODAY'S PRACTICE?

MY INTENTION IS:

AFTER YOGA

TODAY'S PRACTICE INCLUDED:

- ☐ yoga poses (*asana*)
- ☐ breathwork (*pranayama*)
- ☐ meditation (*dhyana*)
- ☐ chanting mantra
- ☐ other: __________

3 WORDS THAT CAPTURE HOW MY PRACTICE WENT:

WHAT STOOD OUT MOST ABOUT TODAY'S PRACTICE?

OTHER THOUGHTS:

BEFORE YOGA

DATE ___/___/___

AFFIRMATION OF THE DAY:

WHAT DO I NEED FROM TODAY'S PRACTICE?

MY INTENTION IS:

AFTER YOGA

TODAY'S PRACTICE INCLUDED:

- ☐ yoga poses (*asana*)
- ☐ breathwork (*pranayama*)
- ☐ meditation (*dhyana*)
- ☐ chanting mantra
- ☐ other: __________

3 WORDS THAT CAPTURE HOW MY PRACTICE WENT:

WHAT AM I MOST PROUD OF?

OTHER THOUGHTS:

BEFORE YOGA

DATE ___/___/___

AFFIRMATION OF THE DAY:

WHAT DO I NEED FROM TODAY'S PRACTICE?

MY INTENTION IS:

AFTER YOGA

TODAY'S PRACTICE INCLUDED:

- ☐ yoga poses (*asana*)
- ☐ breathwork (*pranayama*)
- ☐ meditation (*dhyana*)
- ☐ chanting mantra
- ☐ other: ___

3 WORDS THAT CAPTURE HOW MY PRACTICE WENT:

WHAT WAS THE HARDEST PART OF TODAY'S PRACTICE?

OTHER THOUGHTS:

BEFORE YOGA

DATE ___/___/___

AFFIRMATION OF THE DAY:

WHAT DO I NEED FROM TODAY'S PRACTICE?

MY INTENTION IS:

AFTER YOGA

TODAY'S PRACTICE INCLUDED:

- ☐ yoga poses (*asana*)
- ☐ breathwork (*pranayama*)
- ☐ meditation (*dhyana*)
- ☐ chanting mantra
- ☐ other: ______________

3 WORDS THAT CAPTURE HOW MY PRACTICE WENT:

WHAT DID I LEARN ABOUT MYSELF?

OTHER THOUGHTS:

BEFORE YOGA

DATE ___/___/___

AFFIRMATION OF THE DAY:

WHAT DO I NEED FROM TODAY'S PRACTICE?

MY INTENTION IS:

AFTER YOGA

TODAY'S PRACTICE INCLUDED:

- ☐ yoga poses (*asana*)
- ☐ breathwork (*pranayama*)
- ☐ meditation (*dhyana*)
- ☐ chanting mantra
- ☐ other: ______________

3 WORDS THAT CAPTURE HOW MY PRACTICE WENT:

HOW CAN I TAKE MY YOGA OFF THE MAT AND INTO THE WORLD?

OTHER THOUGHTS:

BEFORE YOGA

DATE ___/___/___

AFFIRMATION OF THE DAY:

WHAT DO I NEED FROM TODAY'S PRACTICE?

MY INTENTION IS:

AFTER YOGA

TODAY'S PRACTICE INCLUDED:

- ☐ yoga poses (*asana*)
- ☐ breathwork (*pranayama*)
- ☐ meditation (*dhyana*)
- ☐ chanting mantra
- ☐ other: ______________

3 WORDS THAT CAPTURE HOW MY PRACTICE WENT:

WHAT DOES YOGA MEAN TO ME?

OTHER THOUGHTS:

BEFORE YOGA

DATE ___/___/___

AFFIRMATION OF THE DAY:

WHAT DO I NEED FROM TODAY'S PRACTICE?

MY INTENTION IS:

AFTER YOGA

TODAY'S PRACTICE INCLUDED:

- ☐ yoga poses (*asana*)
- ☐ breathwork (*pranayama*)
- ☐ meditation (*dhyana*)
- ☐ chanting mantra
- ☐ other: ___

3 WORDS THAT CAPTURE HOW MY PRACTICE WENT:

HOW CONNECTED WAS I TO MY BREATH?

OTHER THOUGHTS:

BEFORE YOGA

DATE ___/___/___

AFFIRMATION OF THE DAY:

WHAT DO I NEED FROM TODAY'S PRACTICE?

MY INTENTION IS:

AFTER YOGA

TODAY'S PRACTICE INCLUDED:

- ☐ yoga poses (*asana*)
- ☐ breathwork (*pranayama*)
- ☐ meditation (*dhyana*)
- ☐ chanting mantra
- ☐ other: __________

3 WORDS THAT CAPTURE HOW MY PRACTICE WENT:

HOW DO I FEEL ABOUT MY BODY RIGHT NOW?

OTHER THOUGHTS:

BEFORE YOGA

DATE ___/___/___

AFFIRMATION OF THE DAY:

WHAT DO I NEED FROM TODAY'S PRACTICE?

MY INTENTION IS:

AFTER YOGA

TODAY'S PRACTICE INCLUDED:

- ☐ yoga poses (*asana*)
- ☐ breathwork (*pranayama*)
- ☐ meditation (*dhyana*)
- ☐ chanting mantra
- ☐ other: ___

3 WORDS THAT CAPTURE HOW MY PRACTICE WENT:

DID I HONOR MY INTENTION DURING PRACTICE?

OTHER THOUGHTS:

BEFORE YOGA

DATE ___/___/___

AFFIRMATION OF THE DAY:

WHAT DO I NEED FROM TODAY'S PRACTICE?

MY INTENTION IS:

AFTER YOGA

TODAY'S PRACTICE INCLUDED:

- ☐ yoga poses (*asana*)
- ☐ breathwork (*pranayama*)
- ☐ meditation (*dhyana*)
- ☐ chanting mantra
- ☐ other: __________

3 WORDS THAT CAPTURE HOW MY PRACTICE WENT:

WHAT WAS THE MAIN EMOTION FELT DURING PRACTICE?

OTHER THOUGHTS:

BEFORE YOGA

DATE ___/___/___

AFFIRMATION OF THE DAY:

____

WHAT DO I NEED FROM TODAY'S PRACTICE?

____

____

____

MY INTENTION IS:

____

____

AFTER YOGA

TODAY'S PRACTICE INCLUDED:

- ☐ yoga poses (*asana*)
- ☐ breathwork (*pranayama*)
- ☐ meditation (*dhyana*)
- ☐ chanting mantra
- ☐ other: _______________

3 WORDS THAT CAPTURE HOW MY PRACTICE WENT:

____

____

____

HOW DO I REACT WHEN FACED WITH A CHALLENGING POSE OR PRACTICE?

____

____

____

OTHER THOUGHTS:

____

____

____

BEFORE YOGA

DATE ___/___/___

AFFIRMATION OF THE DAY:

WHAT DO I NEED FROM TODAY'S PRACTICE?

MY INTENTION IS:

AFTER YOGA

TODAY'S PRACTICE INCLUDED:

- ☐ yoga poses (*asana*)
- ☐ breathwork (*pranayama*)
- ☐ meditation (*dhyana*)
- ☐ chanting mantra
- ☐ other: __________

3 WORDS THAT CAPTURE HOW MY PRACTICE WENT:

HOW ARE EVENTS IN MY LIFE AFFECTING MY PRACTICE?

OTHER THOUGHTS:

BEFORE YOGA

DATE ___/___/___

AFFIRMATION OF THE DAY:

WHAT DO I NEED FROM TODAY'S PRACTICE?

MY INTENTION IS:

AFTER YOGA

TODAY'S PRACTICE INCLUDED:

- ☐ yoga poses (*asana*)
- ☐ breathwork (*pranayama*)
- ☐ meditation (*dhyana*)
- ☐ chanting mantra
- ☐ other: ___

3 WORDS THAT CAPTURE HOW MY PRACTICE WENT:

HOW DOES MY PRACTICE AFFECT MY DAY-TO-DAY LIFE?

OTHER THOUGHTS:

BEFORE YOGA

DATE ___/___/___

AFFIRMATION OF THE DAY:

WHAT DO I NEED FROM TODAY'S PRACTICE?

MY INTENTION IS:

AFTER YOGA

TODAY'S PRACTICE INCLUDED:

- ☐ yoga poses (*asana*)
- ☐ breathwork (*pranayama*)
- ☐ meditation (*dhyana*)
- ☐ chanting mantra
- ☐ other: ______________

3 WORDS THAT CAPTURE HOW MY PRACTICE WENT:

HOW CAN I USE THIS PRACTICE FOR SPIRITUAL GROWTH?

OTHER THOUGHTS:

BEFORE YOGA

DATE ___/___/___

AFFIRMATION OF THE DAY:

WHAT DO I NEED FROM TODAY'S PRACTICE?

MY INTENTION IS:

AFTER YOGA

TODAY'S PRACTICE INCLUDED:

- ☐ yoga poses (*asana*)
- ☐ breathwork (*pranayama*)
- ☐ meditation (*dhyana*)
- ☐ chanting mantra
- ☐ other: __________

3 WORDS THAT CAPTURE HOW MY PRACTICE WENT:

HOW EASY OR DIFFICULT WAS IT FOR ME TO STAY FOCUSED?

OTHER THOUGHTS:

BEFORE YOGA

DATE ___/___/___

AFFIRMATION OF THE DAY:

WHAT DO I NEED FROM TODAY'S PRACTICE?

MY INTENTION IS:

AFTER YOGA

TODAY'S PRACTICE INCLUDED:

- ☐ yoga poses (*asana*)
- ☐ breathwork (*pranayama*)
- ☐ meditation (*dhyana*)
- ☐ chanting mantra
- ☐ other: ___

3 WORDS THAT CAPTURE HOW MY PRACTICE WENT:

WHAT HELPS ME STAY IN THE PRESENT MOMENT?

OTHER THOUGHTS:

BEFORE YOGA

DATE ___/___/___

AFFIRMATION OF THE DAY:

WHAT DO I NEED FROM TODAY'S PRACTICE?

MY INTENTION IS:

AFTER YOGA

TODAY'S PRACTICE INCLUDED:

- ☐ yoga poses (*asana*)
- ☐ breathwork (*pranayama*)
- ☐ meditation (*dhyana*)
- ☐ chanting mantra
- ☐ other: __________

3 WORDS THAT CAPTURE HOW MY PRACTICE WENT:

WHICH TEACHERS DO I FIND MOST INSPIRING AND WHY?

OTHER THOUGHTS:

BEFORE YOGA

DATE ___/___/___

AFFIRMATION OF THE DAY:

WHAT DO I NEED FROM TODAY'S PRACTICE?

MY INTENTION IS:

AFTER YOGA

TODAY'S PRACTICE INCLUDED:

- ☐ yoga poses (*asana*)
- ☐ breathwork (*pranayama*)
- ☐ meditation (*dhyana*)
- ☐ chanting mantra
- ☐ other: ___

3 WORDS THAT CAPTURE HOW MY PRACTICE WENT:

IF I COULD CHANGE ANYTHING FROM TODAY'S PRACTICE, WHAT WOULD IT BE?

OTHER THOUGHTS:

BEFORE YOGA

DATE ___/___/___

AFFIRMATION OF THE DAY:

WHAT DO I NEED FROM TODAY'S PRACTICE?

MY INTENTION IS:

AFTER YOGA

TODAY'S PRACTICE INCLUDED:

- ☐ yoga poses (*asana*)
- ☐ breathwork (*pranayama*)
- ☐ meditation (*dhyana*)
- ☐ chanting mantra
- ☐ other: ___

3 WORDS THAT CAPTURE HOW MY PRACTICE WENT:

DO I TEND TO PUSH TOO HARD OR HOLD BACK?

OTHER THOUGHTS:

BEFORE YOGA

DATE ___/___/___

AFFIRMATION OF THE DAY:

WHAT DO I NEED FROM TODAY'S PRACTICE?

MY INTENTION IS:

AFTER YOGA

TODAY'S PRACTICE INCLUDED:

- ☐ yoga poses (*asana*)
- ☐ breathwork (*pranayama*)
- ☐ meditation (*dhyana*)
- ☐ chanting mantra
- ☐ other: ______

3 WORDS THAT CAPTURE HOW MY PRACTICE WENT:

WHAT MOTIVATES ME TO KEEP PRACTICING EVERY DAY?

OTHER THOUGHTS:

BEFORE YOGA

DATE ___/___/___

AFFIRMATION OF THE DAY:

WHAT DO I NEED FROM TODAY'S PRACTICE?

MY INTENTION IS:

AFTER YOGA

TODAY'S PRACTICE INCLUDED:

- ☐ yoga poses (*asana*)
- ☐ breathwork (*pranayama*)
- ☐ meditation (*dhyana*)
- ☐ chanting mantra
- ☐ other: ___

3 WORDS THAT CAPTURE HOW MY PRACTICE WENT:

HOW HAS MY RELATIONSHIP WITH YOGA CHANGED WITH TIME?

OTHER THOUGHTS:

BEFORE YOGA

DATE ___/___/___

AFFIRMATION OF THE DAY:

WHAT DO I NEED FROM TODAY'S PRACTICE?

MY INTENTION IS:

AFTER YOGA

TODAY'S PRACTICE INCLUDED:

- ☐ yoga poses (*asana*)
- ☐ breathwork (*pranayama*)
- ☐ meditation (*dhyana*)
- ☐ chanting mantra
- ☐ other: ___________

3 WORDS THAT CAPTURE HOW MY PRACTICE WENT:

WHAT DO I NEED MORE OF IN MY PRACTICE?

OTHER THOUGHTS:

BEFORE YOGA

DATE ___/___/___

AFFIRMATION OF THE DAY:

WHAT DO I NEED FROM TODAY'S PRACTICE?

MY INTENTION IS:

AFTER YOGA

TODAY'S PRACTICE INCLUDED:

- ☐ yoga poses (*asana*)
- ☐ breathwork (*pranayama*)
- ☐ meditation (*dhyana*)
- ☐ chanting mantra
- ☐ other: ____________

3 WORDS THAT CAPTURE HOW MY PRACTICE WENT:

WHAT DO I WANT TO WORK ON NEXT TIME?

OTHER THOUGHTS:

BEFORE YOGA

DATE ___/___/___

AFFIRMATION OF THE DAY:

WHAT DO I NEED FROM TODAY'S PRACTICE?

MY INTENTION IS:

AFTER YOGA

TODAY'S PRACTICE INCLUDED:

- ☐ yoga poses (*asana*)
- ☐ breathwork (*pranayama*)
- ☐ meditation (*dhyana*)
- ☐ chanting mantra
- ☐ other: __________

3 WORDS THAT CAPTURE HOW MY PRACTICE WENT:

AM I NEGLECTING AN IMPORTANT ASPECT OF MY YOGA PRACTICE?

OTHER THOUGHTS:

BEFORE YOGA

DATE ___/___/___

AFFIRMATION OF THE DAY:

WHAT DO I NEED FROM TODAY'S PRACTICE?

MY INTENTION IS:

AFTER YOGA

TODAY'S PRACTICE INCLUDED:

- ☐ yoga poses (*asana*)
- ☐ breathwork (*pranayama*)
- ☐ meditation (*dhyana*)
- ☐ chanting mantra
- ☐ other: ___

3 WORDS THAT CAPTURE HOW MY PRACTICE WENT:

DOES MY INTERNAL DIALOGUE TEND TO BE POSITIVE OR NEGATIVE?

OTHER THOUGHTS:

BEFORE YOGA

DATE ___/___/___

AFFIRMATION OF THE DAY:

WHAT DO I NEED FROM TODAY'S PRACTICE?

MY INTENTION IS:

AFTER YOGA

TODAY'S PRACTICE INCLUDED:

- ☐ yoga poses (*asana*)
- ☐ breathwork (*pranayama*)
- ☐ meditation (*dhyana*)
- ☐ chanting mantra
- ☐ other: ____________

3 WORDS THAT CAPTURE HOW MY PRACTICE WENT:

WHAT AM I MOST GRATEFUL FOR RIGHT NOW?

OTHER THOUGHTS:

BEFORE YOGA

DATE ___/___/___

AFFIRMATION OF THE DAY:

WHAT DO I NEED FROM TODAY'S PRACTICE?

MY INTENTION IS:

AFTER YOGA

TODAY'S PRACTICE INCLUDED:

- ☐ yoga poses (*asana*)
- ☐ breathwork (*pranayama*)
- ☐ meditation (*dhyana*)
- ☐ chanting mantra
- ☐ other: ___

3 WORDS THAT CAPTURE HOW MY PRACTICE WENT:

WHAT IS SOMETHING I NEED TO STUDY DEEPER?

OTHER THOUGHTS:

BEFORE YOGA

DATE ___/___/___

AFFIRMATION OF THE DAY:

WHAT DO I NEED FROM TODAY'S PRACTICE?

MY INTENTION IS:

AFTER YOGA

TODAY'S PRACTICE INCLUDED:

- ☐ yoga poses (*asana*)
- ☐ breathwork (*pranayama*)
- ☐ meditation (*dhyana*)
- ☐ chanting mantra
- ☐ other: __________

3 WORDS THAT CAPTURE HOW MY PRACTICE WENT:

HOW DOES YOGA AFFECT MY EMOTIONAL HEALTH?

OTHER THOUGHTS:

BEFORE YOGA

DATE ___/___/___

AFFIRMATION OF THE DAY:

WHAT DO I NEED FROM TODAY'S PRACTICE?

MY INTENTION IS:

AFTER YOGA

TODAY'S PRACTICE INCLUDED:

- ☐ yoga poses (*asana*)
- ☐ breathwork (*pranayama*)
- ☐ meditation (*dhyana*)
- ☐ chanting mantra
- ☐ other: ______________

3 WORDS THAT CAPTURE HOW MY PRACTICE WENT:

HOW DID THIS PRACTICE AFFECT MY ENERGY LEVELS?

OTHER THOUGHTS:

BEFORE YOGA

DATE ___/___/___

AFFIRMATION OF THE DAY:

____

WHAT DO I NEED FROM TODAY'S PRACTICE?

____

____

____

MY INTENTION IS:

____

____

AFTER YOGA

TODAY'S PRACTICE INCLUDED:

- ☐ yoga poses (*asana*)
- ☐ breathwork (*pranayama*)
- ☐ meditation (*dhyana*)
- ☐ chanting mantra
- ☐ other: ______________

3 WORDS THAT CAPTURE HOW MY PRACTICE WENT:

____

____

____

HOW DOES YOGA CONNECT ME WITH MY PURPOSE?

____

____

____

____

OTHER THOUGHTS:

____

____

____

BEFORE YOGA

DATE ___/___/___

AFFIRMATION OF THE DAY:

WHAT DO I NEED FROM TODAY'S PRACTICE?

MY INTENTION IS:

AFTER YOGA

TODAY'S PRACTICE INCLUDED:

- ☐ yoga poses (*asana*)
- ☐ breathwork (*pranayama*)
- ☐ meditation (*dhyana*)
- ☐ chanting mantra
- ☐ other: __________

3 WORDS THAT CAPTURE HOW MY PRACTICE WENT:

WHAT STOOD OUT MOST ABOUT TODAY'S PRACTICE?

OTHER THOUGHTS:

BEFORE YOGA

DATE ___/___/___

AFFIRMATION OF THE DAY:

WHAT DO I NEED FROM TODAY'S PRACTICE?

MY INTENTION IS:

AFTER YOGA

TODAY'S PRACTICE INCLUDED:

- ☐ yoga poses (*asana*)
- ☐ breathwork (*pranayama*)
- ☐ meditation (*dhyana*)
- ☐ chanting mantra
- ☐ other: ____________

3 WORDS THAT CAPTURE HOW MY PRACTICE WENT:

WHAT AM I MOST PROUD OF?

OTHER THOUGHTS:

BEFORE YOGA

DATE ___/___/___

AFFIRMATION OF THE DAY:

WHAT DO I NEED FROM TODAY'S PRACTICE?

MY INTENTION IS:

AFTER YOGA

TODAY'S PRACTICE INCLUDED:

- ☐ yoga poses (*asana*)
- ☐ breathwork (*pranayama*)
- ☐ meditation (*dhyana*)
- ☐ chanting mantra
- ☐ other: ______________

3 WORDS THAT CAPTURE HOW MY PRACTICE WENT:

WHAT WAS THE HARDEST PART OF TODAY'S PRACTICE?

OTHER THOUGHTS:

BEFORE YOGA

DATE ___/___/___

AFFIRMATION OF THE DAY:

WHAT DO I NEED FROM TODAY'S PRACTICE?

MY INTENTION IS:

AFTER YOGA

TODAY'S PRACTICE INCLUDED:

- ☐ yoga poses (*asana*)
- ☐ breathwork (*pranayama*)
- ☐ meditation (*dhyana*)
- ☐ chanting mantra
- ☐ other: __________

3 WORDS THAT CAPTURE HOW MY PRACTICE WENT:

WHAT DID I LEARN ABOUT MYSELF?

OTHER THOUGHTS:

BEFORE YOGA

DATE ___/___/___

AFFIRMATION OF THE DAY:

WHAT DO I NEED FROM TODAY'S PRACTICE?

MY INTENTION IS:

AFTER YOGA

TODAY'S PRACTICE INCLUDED:

- ☐ yoga poses (*asana*)
- ☐ breathwork (*pranayama*)
- ☐ meditation (*dhyana*)
- ☐ chanting mantra
- ☐ other:

3 WORDS THAT CAPTURE HOW MY PRACTICE WENT:

HOW CAN I TAKE MY YOGA OFF THE MAT AND INTO THE WORLD?

OTHER THOUGHTS:

BEFORE YOGA

DATE ___/___/___

AFFIRMATION OF THE DAY:

WHAT DO I NEED FROM TODAY'S PRACTICE?

MY INTENTION IS:

AFTER YOGA

TODAY'S PRACTICE INCLUDED:

- ☐ yoga poses (*asana*)
- ☐ breathwork (*pranayama*)
- ☐ meditation (*dhyana*)
- ☐ chanting mantra
- ☐ other: ____________

3 WORDS THAT CAPTURE HOW MY PRACTICE WENT:

WHAT DOES YOGA MEAN TO ME?

OTHER THOUGHTS:

BEFORE YOGA

DATE ___/___/___

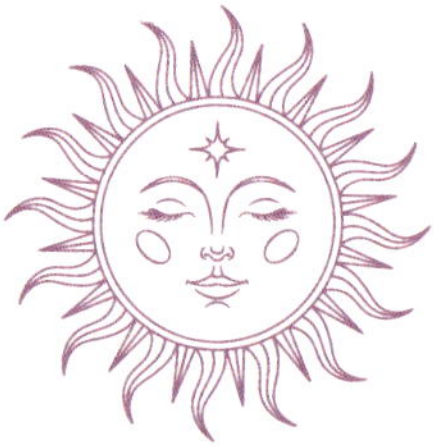

AFFIRMATION OF THE DAY:

WHAT DO I NEED FROM TODAY'S PRACTICE?

MY INTENTION IS:

AFTER YOGA

TODAY'S PRACTICE INCLUDED:

- ☐ yoga poses (*asana*)
- ☐ breathwork (*pranayama*)
- ☐ meditation (*dhyana*)
- ☐ chanting mantra
- ☐ other: ____________

3 WORDS THAT CAPTURE HOW MY PRACTICE WENT:

HOW CONNECTED WAS I TO MY BREATH?

OTHER THOUGHTS:

BEFORE YOGA

DATE ___/___/___

AFFIRMATION OF THE DAY:

WHAT DO I NEED FROM TODAY'S PRACTICE?

MY INTENTION IS:

AFTER YOGA

TODAY'S PRACTICE INCLUDED:

- ☐ yoga poses (*asana*)
- ☐ breathwork (*pranayama*)
- ☐ meditation (*dhyana*)
- ☐ chanting mantra
- ☐ other: ______________

3 WORDS THAT CAPTURE HOW MY PRACTICE WENT:

HOW DO I FEEL ABOUT MY BODY RIGHT NOW?

OTHER THOUGHTS:

BEFORE YOGA

DATE ___/___/___

AFFIRMATION OF THE DAY:

WHAT DO I NEED FROM TODAY'S PRACTICE?

MY INTENTION IS:

AFTER YOGA

TODAY'S PRACTICE INCLUDED:

- ☐ yoga poses (*asana*)
- ☐ breathwork (*pranayama*)
- ☐ meditation (*dhyana*)
- ☐ chanting mantra
- ☐ other: ________

3 WORDS THAT CAPTURE HOW MY PRACTICE WENT:

DID I HONOR MY INTENTION DURING PRACTICE?

OTHER THOUGHTS:

BEFORE YOGA

DATE ___/___/___

AFFIRMATION OF THE DAY:

WHAT DO I NEED FROM TODAY'S PRACTICE?

MY INTENTION IS:

AFTER YOGA

TODAY'S PRACTICE INCLUDED:

- ☐ yoga poses (*asana*)
- ☐ breathwork (*pranayama*)
- ☐ meditation (*dhyana*)
- ☐ chanting mantra
- ☐ other: ___

3 WORDS THAT CAPTURE HOW MY PRACTICE WENT:

WHAT WAS THE MAIN EMOTION FELT DURING PRACTICE?

OTHER THOUGHTS:

BEFORE YOGA

DATE ___/___/___

AFFIRMATION OF THE DAY:

WHAT DO I NEED FROM TODAY'S PRACTICE?

MY INTENTION IS:

AFTER YOGA

TODAY'S PRACTICE INCLUDED:

- ☐ yoga poses (*asana*)
- ☐ breathwork (*pranayama*)
- ☐ meditation (*dhyana*)
- ☐ chanting mantra
- ☐ other: ___

3 WORDS THAT CAPTURE HOW MY PRACTICE WENT:

HOW DO I REACT WHEN FACED WITH A CHALLENGING POSE OR PRACTICE?

OTHER THOUGHTS:

BEFORE YOGA

DATE ___/___/___

AFFIRMATION OF THE DAY:

WHAT DO I NEED FROM TODAY'S PRACTICE?

MY INTENTION IS:

AFTER YOGA

TODAY'S PRACTICE INCLUDED:

- ☐ yoga poses (*asana*)
- ☐ breathwork (*pranayama*)
- ☐ meditation (*dhyana*)
- ☐ chanting mantra
- ☐ other: ______________

3 WORDS THAT CAPTURE HOW MY PRACTICE WENT:

HOW ARE EVENTS IN MY LIFE AFFECTING MY PRACTICE?

OTHER THOUGHTS:

BEFORE YOGA

DATE ___/___/___

AFFIRMATION OF THE DAY:

WHAT DO I NEED FROM TODAY'S PRACTICE?

MY INTENTION IS:

AFTER YOGA

TODAY'S PRACTICE INCLUDED:

- ☐ yoga poses (*asana*)
- ☐ breathwork (*pranayama*)
- ☐ meditation (*dhyana*)
- ☐ chanting mantra
- ☐ other: ________

3 WORDS THAT CAPTURE HOW MY PRACTICE WENT:

HOW DOES MY PRACTICE AFFECT MY DAY-TO-DAY LIFE?

OTHER THOUGHTS:

BEFORE YOGA

DATE ___/___/___

AFFIRMATION OF THE DAY:

WHAT DO I NEED FROM TODAY'S PRACTICE?

MY INTENTION IS:

AFTER YOGA

TODAY'S PRACTICE INCLUDED:

- ☐ yoga poses (*asana*)
- ☐ breathwork (*pranayama*)
- ☐ meditation (*dhyana*)
- ☐ chanting mantra
- ☐ other: ___

3 WORDS THAT CAPTURE HOW MY PRACTICE WENT:

HOW CAN I USE THIS PRACTICE FOR SPIRITUAL GROWTH?

OTHER THOUGHTS:

BEFORE YOGA

DATE ___/___/___

AFFIRMATION OF THE DAY:

WHAT DO I NEED FROM TODAY'S PRACTICE?

MY INTENTION IS:

AFTER YOGA

TODAY'S PRACTICE INCLUDED:

- ☐ yoga poses (*asana*)
- ☐ breathwork (*pranayama*)
- ☐ meditation (*dhyana*)
- ☐ chanting mantra
- ☐ other: ___

3 WORDS THAT CAPTURE HOW MY PRACTICE WENT:

HOW EASY OR DIFFICULT WAS IT FOR ME TO STAY FOCUSED?

OTHER THOUGHTS:

BEFORE YOGA

DATE ___/___/___

AFFIRMATION OF THE DAY:

WHAT DO I NEED FROM TODAY'S PRACTICE?

MY INTENTION IS:

AFTER YOGA

TODAY'S PRACTICE INCLUDED:

- ☐ yoga poses (*asana*)
- ☐ breathwork (*pranayama*)
- ☐ meditation (*dhyana*)
- ☐ chanting mantra
- ☐ other: ___

3 WORDS THAT CAPTURE HOW MY PRACTICE WENT:

WHAT HELPS ME STAY IN THE PRESENT MOMENT?

OTHER THOUGHTS:

BEFORE YOGA

DATE ___/___/___

AFFIRMATION OF THE DAY:

WHAT DO I NEED FROM TODAY'S PRACTICE?

MY INTENTION IS:

AFTER YOGA

TODAY'S PRACTICE INCLUDED:

- ☐ yoga poses (*asana*)
- ☐ breathwork (*pranayama*)
- ☐ meditation (*dhyana*)
- ☐ chanting mantra
- ☐ other: ______________

3 WORDS THAT CAPTURE HOW MY PRACTICE WENT:

WHICH TEACHERS DO I FIND MOST INSPIRING AND WHY?

OTHER THOUGHTS:

BEFORE YOGA

DATE ___/___/___

AFFIRMATION OF THE DAY:

WHAT DO I NEED FROM TODAY'S PRACTICE?

MY INTENTION IS:

AFTER YOGA

TODAY'S PRACTICE INCLUDED:

- ☐ yoga poses (*asana*)
- ☐ breathwork (*pranayama*)
- ☐ meditation (*dhyana*)
- ☐ chanting mantra
- ☐ other: ___

3 WORDS THAT CAPTURE HOW MY PRACTICE WENT:

IF I COULD CHANGE ANYTHING FROM TODAY'S PRACTICE, WHAT WOULD IT BE?

OTHER THOUGHTS:

BEFORE YOGA

DATE ___/___/___

AFFIRMATION OF THE DAY:

WHAT DO I NEED FROM TODAY'S PRACTICE?

MY INTENTION IS:

AFTER YOGA

TODAY'S PRACTICE INCLUDED:

- ☐ yoga poses (*asana*)
- ☐ breathwork (*pranayama*)
- ☐ meditation (*dhyana*)
- ☐ chanting mantra
- ☐ other: ______________

3 WORDS THAT CAPTURE HOW MY PRACTICE WENT:

DO I TEND TO PUSH TOO HARD OR HOLD BACK?

OTHER THOUGHTS:

BEFORE YOGA

DATE ___/___/___

AFFIRMATION OF THE DAY:

WHAT DO I NEED FROM TODAY'S PRACTICE?

MY INTENTION IS:

AFTER YOGA

TODAY'S PRACTICE INCLUDED:

- ☐ yoga poses (*asana*)
- ☐ breathwork (*pranayama*)
- ☐ meditation (*dhyana*)
- ☐ chanting mantra
- ☐ other: ____________

3 WORDS THAT CAPTURE HOW MY PRACTICE WENT:

WHAT MOTIVATES ME TO KEEP PRACTICING EVERY DAY?

OTHER THOUGHTS:

BEFORE YOGA

DATE ___/___/___

AFFIRMATION OF THE DAY:

WHAT DO I NEED FROM TODAY'S PRACTICE?

MY INTENTION IS:

AFTER YOGA

TODAY'S PRACTICE INCLUDED:

- ☐ yoga poses (*asana*)
- ☐ breathwork (*pranayama*)
- ☐ meditation (*dhyana*)
- ☐ chanting mantra
- ☐ other: ___________

3 WORDS THAT CAPTURE HOW MY PRACTICE WENT:

HOW HAS MY RELATIONSHIP WITH YOGA CHANGED WITH TIME?

OTHER THOUGHTS:

BEFORE YOGA

DATE ___/___/___

AFFIRMATION OF THE DAY:

WHAT DO I NEED FROM TODAY'S PRACTICE?

MY INTENTION IS:

AFTER YOGA

TODAY'S PRACTICE INCLUDED:

- ☐ yoga poses (*asana*)
- ☐ breathwork (*pranayama*)
- ☐ meditation (*dhyana*)
- ☐ chanting mantra
- ☐ other: ____________

3 WORDS THAT CAPTURE HOW MY PRACTICE WENT:

WHAT DO I NEED MORE OF IN MY PRACTICE?

OTHER THOUGHTS:

BEFORE YOGA

DATE ___/___/___

AFFIRMATION OF THE DAY:

WHAT DO I NEED FROM TODAY'S PRACTICE?

MY INTENTION IS:

AFTER YOGA

TODAY'S PRACTICE INCLUDED:

- ☐ yoga poses (*asana*)
- ☐ breathwork (*pranayama*)
- ☐ meditation (*dhyana*)
- ☐ chanting mantra
- ☐ other: ____________

3 WORDS THAT CAPTURE HOW MY PRACTICE WENT:

WHAT DO I WANT TO WORK ON NEXT TIME?

OTHER THOUGHTS:

BEFORE YOGA

DATE ___/___/___

AFFIRMATION OF THE DAY:

WHAT DO I NEED FROM TODAY'S PRACTICE?

MY INTENTION IS:

AFTER YOGA

TODAY'S PRACTICE INCLUDED:

- ☐ yoga poses (*asana*)
- ☐ breathwork (*pranayama*)
- ☐ meditation (*dhyana*)
- ☐ chanting mantra
- ☐ other: __________

3 WORDS THAT CAPTURE HOW MY PRACTICE WENT:

AM I NEGLECTING AN IMPORTANT ASPECT OF MY YOGA PRACTICE?

OTHER THOUGHTS:

BEFORE YOGA

DATE ___/___/___

AFFIRMATION OF THE DAY:

WHAT DO I NEED FROM TODAY'S PRACTICE?

MY INTENTION IS:

AFTER YOGA

TODAY'S PRACTICE INCLUDED:

- ☐ yoga poses (*asana*)
- ☐ breathwork (*pranayama*)
- ☐ meditation (*dhyana*)
- ☐ chanting mantra
- ☐ other: ______________

3 WORDS THAT CAPTURE HOW MY PRACTICE WENT:

DOES MY INTERNAL DIALOGUE TEND TO BE POSITIVE OR NEGATIVE?

OTHER THOUGHTS:

BEFORE YOGA

DATE ___/___/___

AFFIRMATION OF THE DAY:

WHAT DO I NEED FROM TODAY'S PRACTICE?

MY INTENTION IS:

AFTER YOGA

TODAY'S PRACTICE INCLUDED:

- ☐ yoga poses (*asana*)
- ☐ breathwork (*pranayama*)
- ☐ meditation (*dhyana*)
- ☐ chanting mantra
- ☐ other: ____________

3 WORDS THAT CAPTURE HOW MY PRACTICE WENT:

WHAT AM I MOST GRATEFUL FOR RIGHT NOW?

OTHER THOUGHTS:

BEFORE YOGA

DATE ___/___/___

AFFIRMATION OF THE DAY:

WHAT DO I NEED FROM TODAY'S PRACTICE?

MY INTENTION IS:

AFTER YOGA

TODAY'S PRACTICE INCLUDED:

- ☐ yoga poses (*asana*)
- ☐ breathwork (*pranayama*)
- ☐ meditation (*dhyana*)
- ☐ chanting mantra
- ☐ other: ___

3 WORDS THAT CAPTURE HOW MY PRACTICE WENT:

WHAT IS SOMETHING I NEED TO STUDY DEEPER?

OTHER THOUGHTS:

BEFORE YOGA

DATE ___/___/___

AFFIRMATION OF THE DAY:

WHAT DO I NEED FROM TODAY'S PRACTICE?

MY INTENTION IS:

AFTER YOGA

TODAY'S PRACTICE INCLUDED:

- ☐ yoga poses (*asana*)
- ☐ breathwork (*pranayama*)
- ☐ meditation (*dhyana*)
- ☐ chanting mantra
- ☐ other: ___

3 WORDS THAT CAPTURE HOW MY PRACTICE WENT:

HOW DOES YOGA AFFECT MY EMOTIONAL HEALTH?

OTHER THOUGHTS:

BEFORE YOGA

DATE ___/___/___

AFFIRMATION OF THE DAY:

WHAT DO I NEED FROM TODAY'S PRACTICE?

MY INTENTION IS:

AFTER YOGA

TODAY'S PRACTICE INCLUDED:

- ☐ yoga poses (*asana*)
- ☐ breathwork (*pranayama*)
- ☐ meditation (*dhyana*)
- ☐ chanting mantra
- ☐ other: ______

3 WORDS THAT CAPTURE HOW MY PRACTICE WENT:

HOW DID THIS PRACTICE AFFECT MY ENERGY LEVELS?

OTHER THOUGHTS:

BEFORE YOGA

DATE ___/___/___

AFFIRMATION OF THE DAY:

WHAT DO I NEED FROM TODAY'S PRACTICE?

MY INTENTION IS:

AFTER YOGA

TODAY'S PRACTICE INCLUDED:

- ☐ yoga poses (*asana*)
- ☐ breathwork (*pranayama*)
- ☐ meditation (*dhyana*)
- ☐ chanting mantra
- ☐ other: ___________

3 WORDS THAT CAPTURE HOW MY PRACTICE WENT:

HOW DOES YOGA CONNECT ME WITH MY PURPOSE?

OTHER THOUGHTS:

BEFORE YOGA

DATE ___/___/___

AFFIRMATION OF THE DAY:

WHAT DO I NEED FROM TODAY'S PRACTICE?

MY INTENTION IS:

AFTER YOGA

TODAY'S PRACTICE INCLUDED:

- ☐ yoga poses (*asana*)
- ☐ breathwork (*pranayama*)
- ☐ meditation (*dhyana*)
- ☐ chanting mantra
- ☐ other: ______________

3 WORDS THAT CAPTURE HOW MY PRACTICE WENT:

WHAT STOOD OUT MOST ABOUT TODAY'S PRACTICE?

OTHER THOUGHTS:

BEFORE YOGA

DATE ___/___/___

AFFIRMATION OF THE DAY:

WHAT DO I NEED FROM TODAY'S PRACTICE?

MY INTENTION IS:

AFTER YOGA

TODAY'S PRACTICE INCLUDED:

- ☐ yoga poses (*asana*)
- ☐ breathwork (*pranayama*)
- ☐ meditation (*dhyana*)
- ☐ chanting mantra
- ☐ other: ______________

3 WORDS THAT CAPTURE HOW MY PRACTICE WENT:

WHAT AM I MOST PROUD OF?

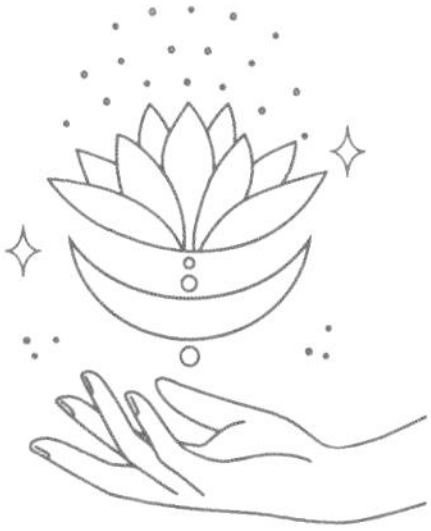

OTHER THOUGHTS:

BEFORE YOGA

DATE ___/___/___

AFFIRMATION OF THE DAY:

WHAT DO I NEED FROM TODAY'S PRACTICE?

MY INTENTION IS:

AFTER YOGA

TODAY'S PRACTICE INCLUDED:

- ☐ yoga poses (*asana*)
- ☐ breathwork (*pranayama*)
- ☐ meditation (*dhyana*)
- ☐ chanting mantra
- ☐ other: __________

3 WORDS THAT CAPTURE HOW MY PRACTICE WENT:

WHAT WAS THE HARDEST PART OF TODAY'S PRACTICE?

OTHER THOUGHTS:

BEFORE YOGA

DATE ___/___/___

AFFIRMATION OF THE DAY:

WHAT DO I NEED FROM TODAY'S PRACTICE?

MY INTENTION IS:

AFTER YOGA

TODAY'S PRACTICE INCLUDED:

- ☐ yoga poses (*asana*)
- ☐ breathwork (*pranayama*)
- ☐ meditation (*dhyana*)
- ☐ chanting mantra
- ☐ other: ___

3 WORDS THAT CAPTURE HOW MY PRACTICE WENT:

WHAT DID I LEARN ABOUT MYSELF?

OTHER THOUGHTS:

BEFORE YOGA

DATE ___/___/___

AFFIRMATION OF THE DAY:

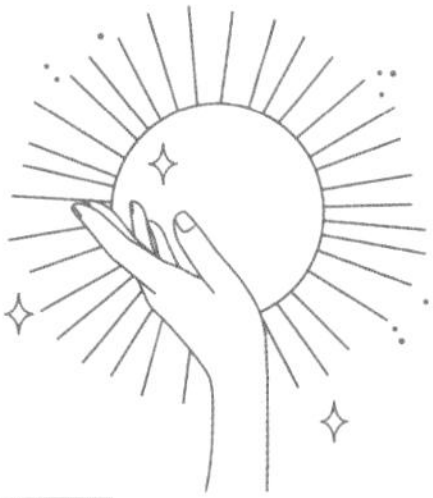

WHAT DO I NEED FROM TODAY'S PRACTICE?

MY INTENTION IS:

AFTER YOGA

TODAY'S PRACTICE INCLUDED:

- ☐ yoga poses (*asana*)
- ☐ breathwork (*pranayama*)
- ☐ meditation (*dhyana*)
- ☐ chanting mantra
- ☐ other: ___

3 WORDS THAT CAPTURE HOW MY PRACTICE WENT:

HOW CAN I TAKE MY YOGA OFF THE MAT AND INTO THE WORLD?

OTHER THOUGHTS:

BEFORE YOGA

DATE ___/___/___

AFFIRMATION OF THE DAY:

WHAT DO I NEED FROM TODAY'S PRACTICE?

MY INTENTION IS:

AFTER YOGA

TODAY'S PRACTICE INCLUDED:

- ☐ yoga poses (*asana*)
- ☐ breathwork (*pranayama*)
- ☐ meditation (*dhyana*)
- ☐ chanting mantra
- ☐ other: ___________

3 WORDS THAT CAPTURE HOW MY PRACTICE WENT:

WHAT DOES YOGA MEAN TO ME?

OTHER THOUGHTS:

BEFORE YOGA

DATE ___/___/___

AFFIRMATION OF THE DAY:

WHAT DO I NEED FROM TODAY'S PRACTICE?

MY INTENTION IS:

AFTER YOGA

TODAY'S PRACTICE INCLUDED:

- ☐ yoga poses (*asana*)
- ☐ breathwork (*pranayama*)
- ☐ meditation (*dhyana*)
- ☐ chanting mantra
- ☐ other: __________

3 WORDS THAT CAPTURE HOW MY PRACTICE WENT:

HOW CONNECTED WAS I TO MY BREATH?

OTHER THOUGHTS:

BEFORE YOGA

DATE ___/___/___

AFFIRMATION OF THE DAY:

WHAT DO I NEED FROM TODAY'S PRACTICE?

MY INTENTION IS:

AFTER YOGA

TODAY'S PRACTICE INCLUDED:

- ☐ yoga poses (*asana*)
- ☐ breathwork (*pranayama*)
- ☐ meditation (*dhyana*)
- ☐ chanting mantra
- ☐ other: ________

3 WORDS THAT CAPTURE HOW MY PRACTICE WENT:

HOW DO I FEEL ABOUT MY BODY RIGHT NOW?

OTHER THOUGHTS:

BEFORE YOGA

DATE ___/___/___

AFFIRMATION OF THE DAY:

WHAT DO I NEED FROM TODAY'S PRACTICE?

MY INTENTION IS:

AFTER YOGA

TODAY'S PRACTICE INCLUDED:

- ☐ yoga poses (*asana*)
- ☐ breathwork (*pranayama*)
- ☐ meditation (*dhyana*)
- ☐ chanting mantra
- ☐ other: ___

3 WORDS THAT CAPTURE HOW MY PRACTICE WENT:

DID I HONOR MY INTENTION DURING PRACTICE?

OTHER THOUGHTS:

BEFORE YOGA

DATE ___/___/___

AFFIRMATION OF THE DAY:

WHAT DO I NEED FROM TODAY'S PRACTICE?

MY INTENTION IS:

AFTER YOGA

TODAY'S PRACTICE INCLUDED:

- ☐ yoga poses (*asana*)
- ☐ breathwork (*pranayama*)
- ☐ meditation (*dhyana*)
- ☐ chanting mantra
- ☐ other: __________

3 WORDS THAT CAPTURE HOW MY PRACTICE WENT:

WHAT WAS THE MAIN EMOTION FELT DURING PRACTICE?

OTHER THOUGHTS:

BEFORE YOGA

DATE ___/___/___

AFFIRMATION OF THE DAY:

WHAT DO I NEED FROM TODAY'S PRACTICE?

MY INTENTION IS:

AFTER YOGA

TODAY'S PRACTICE INCLUDED:

- ☐ yoga poses (*asana*)
- ☐ breathwork (*pranayama*)
- ☐ meditation (*dhyana*)
- ☐ chanting mantra
- ☐ other: ______

3 WORDS THAT CAPTURE HOW MY PRACTICE WENT:

HOW DO I REACT WHEN FACED WITH A CHALLENGING POSE OR PRACTICE?

OTHER THOUGHTS:

BEFORE YOGA

DATE ___/___/___

AFFIRMATION OF THE DAY:

WHAT DO I NEED FROM TODAY'S PRACTICE?

MY INTENTION IS:

AFTER YOGA

TODAY'S PRACTICE INCLUDED:

- ☐ yoga poses (*asana*)
- ☐ breathwork (*pranayama*)
- ☐ meditation (*dhyana*)
- ☐ chanting mantra
- ☐ other: ___

3 WORDS THAT CAPTURE HOW MY PRACTICE WENT:

HOW ARE EVENTS IN MY LIFE AFFECTING MY PRACTICE?

OTHER THOUGHTS:

BEFORE YOGA

DATE ___/___/___

AFFIRMATION OF THE DAY:

WHAT DO I NEED FROM TODAY'S PRACTICE?

MY INTENTION IS:

AFTER YOGA

TODAY'S PRACTICE INCLUDED:

- ☐ yoga poses (*asana*)
- ☐ breathwork (*pranayama*)
- ☐ meditation (*dhyana*)
- ☐ chanting mantra
- ☐ other: __________

3 WORDS THAT CAPTURE HOW MY PRACTICE WENT:

HOW DOES MY PRACTICE AFFECT MY DAY-TO-DAY LIFE?

OTHER THOUGHTS:

BEFORE YOGA

DATE ___/___/___

AFFIRMATION OF THE DAY:

WHAT DO I NEED FROM TODAY'S PRACTICE?

MY INTENTION IS:

AFTER YOGA

TODAY'S PRACTICE INCLUDED:

- ☐ yoga poses (*asana*)
- ☐ breathwork (*pranayama*)
- ☐ meditation (*dhyana*)
- ☐ chanting mantra
- ☐ other: ___

3 WORDS THAT CAPTURE HOW MY PRACTICE WENT:

HOW CAN I USE THIS PRACTICE FOR SPIRITUAL GROWTH?

OTHER THOUGHTS:

BEFORE YOGA

DATE ___/___/___

AFFIRMATION OF THE DAY:

WHAT DO I NEED FROM TODAY'S PRACTICE?

MY INTENTION IS:

AFTER YOGA

TODAY'S PRACTICE INCLUDED:

- ☐ yoga poses (*asana*)
- ☐ breathwork (*pranayama*)
- ☐ meditation (*dhyana*)
- ☐ chanting mantra
- ☐ other: ___

3 WORDS THAT CAPTURE HOW MY PRACTICE WENT:

HOW EASY OR DIFFICULT WAS IT FOR ME TO STAY FOCUSED?

OTHER THOUGHTS:

BEFORE YOGA

DATE ___/___/___

AFFIRMATION OF THE DAY:

WHAT DO I NEED FROM TODAY'S PRACTICE?

MY INTENTION IS:

AFTER YOGA

TODAY'S PRACTICE INCLUDED:

- ☐ yoga poses (*asana*)
- ☐ breathwork (*pranayama*)
- ☐ meditation (*dhyana*)
- ☐ chanting mantra
- ☐ other: ____________

3 WORDS THAT CAPTURE HOW MY PRACTICE WENT:

WHAT HELPS ME STAY IN THE PRESENT MOMENT?

OTHER THOUGHTS:

BEFORE YOGA

DATE ___/___/___

AFFIRMATION OF THE DAY:

WHAT DO I NEED FROM TODAY'S PRACTICE?

MY INTENTION IS:

AFTER YOGA

TODAY'S PRACTICE INCLUDED:

- ☐ yoga poses (*asana*)
- ☐ breathwork (*pranayama*)
- ☐ meditation (*dhyana*)
- ☐ chanting mantra
- ☐ other: __________

3 WORDS THAT CAPTURE HOW MY PRACTICE WENT:

WHICH TEACHERS DO I FIND MOST INSPIRING AND WHY?

OTHER THOUGHTS:

BEFORE YOGA

DATE ___/___/___

AFFIRMATION OF THE DAY:

WHAT DO I NEED FROM TODAY'S PRACTICE?

MY INTENTION IS:

AFTER YOGA

TODAY'S PRACTICE INCLUDED:

- ☐ yoga poses (*asana*)
- ☐ breathwork (*pranayama*)
- ☐ meditation (*dhyana*)
- ☐ chanting mantra
- ☐ other: ______________

3 WORDS THAT CAPTURE HOW MY PRACTICE WENT:

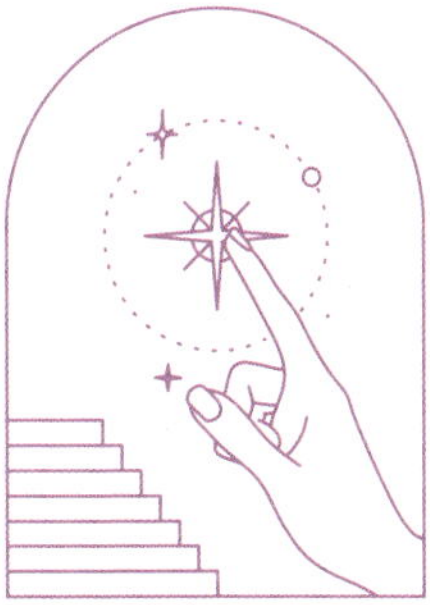

IF I COULD CHANGE ANYTHING FROM TODAY'S PRACTICE, WHAT WOULD IT BE?

OTHER THOUGHTS:

BEFORE YOGA

DATE ____/____/____

AFFIRMATION OF THE DAY:

WHAT DO I NEED FROM TODAY'S PRACTICE?

MY INTENTION IS:

AFTER YOGA

TODAY'S PRACTICE INCLUDED:

- ☐ yoga poses (*asana*)
- ☐ breathwork (*pranayama*)
- ☐ meditation (*dhyana*)
- ☐ chanting mantra
- ☐ other: ________________

3 WORDS THAT CAPTURE HOW MY PRACTICE WENT:

DO I TEND TO PUSH TOO HARD OR HOLD BACK?

OTHER THOUGHTS:

BEFORE YOGA

DATE ___/___/___

AFFIRMATION OF THE DAY:

WHAT DO I NEED FROM TODAY'S PRACTICE?

MY INTENTION IS:

AFTER YOGA

TODAY'S PRACTICE INCLUDED:

- ☐ yoga poses (*asana*)
- ☐ breathwork (*pranayama*)
- ☐ meditation (*dhyana*)
- ☐ chanting mantra
- ☐ other: ___

3 WORDS THAT CAPTURE HOW MY PRACTICE WENT:

WHAT MOTIVATES ME TO KEEP PRACTICING EVERY DAY?

OTHER THOUGHTS:

BEFORE YOGA

DATE ___/___/___

AFFIRMATION OF THE DAY:

WHAT DO I NEED FROM TODAY'S PRACTICE?

MY INTENTION IS:

AFTER YOGA

TODAY'S PRACTICE INCLUDED:

- ☐ yoga poses (*asana*)
- ☐ breathwork (*pranayama*)
- ☐ meditation (*dhyana*)
- ☐ chanting mantra
- ☐ other: ___________

3 WORDS THAT CAPTURE HOW MY PRACTICE WENT:

HOW HAS MY RELATIONSHIP WITH YOGA CHANGED WITH TIME?

OTHER THOUGHTS:

BEFORE YOGA

DATE ___/___/___

AFFIRMATION OF THE DAY:

WHAT DO I NEED FROM TODAY'S PRACTICE?

MY INTENTION IS:

AFTER YOGA

TODAY'S PRACTICE INCLUDED:

- ☐ yoga poses (*asana*)
- ☐ breathwork (*pranayama*)
- ☐ meditation (*dhyana*)
- ☐ chanting mantra
- ☐ other: ______________

3 WORDS THAT CAPTURE HOW MY PRACTICE WENT:

WHAT DO I NEED MORE OF IN MY PRACTICE?

OTHER THOUGHTS:

BEFORE YOGA

DATE ___/___/___

AFFIRMATION OF THE DAY:

WHAT DO I NEED FROM TODAY'S PRACTICE?

MY INTENTION IS:

AFTER YOGA

TODAY'S PRACTICE INCLUDED:

- ☐ yoga poses (*asana*)
- ☐ breathwork (*pranayama*)
- ☐ meditation (*dhyana*)
- ☐ chanting mantra
- ☐ other: __________

3 WORDS THAT CAPTURE HOW MY PRACTICE WENT:

WHAT DO I WANT TO WORK ON NEXT TIME?

OTHER THOUGHTS:

BEFORE YOGA

DATE ___/___/___

AFFIRMATION OF THE DAY:

WHAT DO I NEED FROM TODAY'S PRACTICE?

MY INTENTION IS:

AFTER YOGA

TODAY'S PRACTICE INCLUDED:

- ☐ yoga poses (*asana*)
- ☐ breathwork (*pranayama*)
- ☐ meditation (*dhyana*)
- ☐ chanting mantra
- ☐ other: ______________

3 WORDS THAT CAPTURE HOW MY PRACTICE WENT:

AM I NEGLECTING AN IMPORTANT ASPECT OF MY YOGA PRACTICE?

OTHER THOUGHTS:

BEFORE YOGA

DATE ___/___/___

AFFIRMATION OF THE DAY:

WHAT DO I NEED FROM TODAY'S PRACTICE?

MY INTENTION IS:

AFTER YOGA

TODAY'S PRACTICE INCLUDED:

- ☐ yoga poses (*asana*)
- ☐ breathwork (*pranayama*)
- ☐ meditation (*dhyana*)
- ☐ chanting mantra
- ☐ other: ______

3 WORDS THAT CAPTURE HOW MY PRACTICE WENT:

DOES MY INTERNAL DIALOGUE TEND TO BE POSITIVE OR NEGATIVE?

OTHER THOUGHTS:

BEFORE YOGA

DATE ___/___/___

AFFIRMATION OF THE DAY:

WHAT DO I NEED FROM TODAY'S PRACTICE?

MY INTENTION IS:

AFTER YOGA

TODAY'S PRACTICE INCLUDED:

- ☐ yoga poses (*asana*)
- ☐ breathwork (*pranayama*)
- ☐ meditation (*dhyana*)
- ☐ chanting mantra
- ☐ other: ______

3 WORDS THAT CAPTURE HOW MY PRACTICE WENT:

WHAT AM I MOST GRATEFUL FOR RIGHT NOW?

OTHER THOUGHTS:

BEFORE YOGA

DATE ___/___/___

AFFIRMATION OF THE DAY:

WHAT DO I NEED FROM TODAY'S PRACTICE?

MY INTENTION IS:

AFTER YOGA

TODAY'S PRACTICE INCLUDED:

- ☐ yoga poses (*asana*)
- ☐ breathwork (*pranayama*)
- ☐ meditation (*dhyana*)
- ☐ chanting mantra
- ☐ other: ___

3 WORDS THAT CAPTURE HOW MY PRACTICE WENT:

WHAT IS SOMETHING I NEED TO STUDY DEEPER?

OTHER THOUGHTS:

BEFORE YOGA

DATE ___/___/___

AFFIRMATION OF THE DAY:

WHAT DO I NEED FROM TODAY'S PRACTICE?

MY INTENTION IS:

AFTER YOGA

TODAY'S PRACTICE INCLUDED:

- ☐ yoga poses (*asana*)
- ☐ breathwork (*pranayama*)
- ☐ meditation (*dhyana*)
- ☐ chanting mantra
- ☐ other: __________

3 WORDS THAT CAPTURE HOW MY PRACTICE WENT:

HOW DOES YOGA AFFECT MY EMOTIONAL HEALTH?

OTHER THOUGHTS:

BEFORE YOGA

DATE ___/___/___

AFFIRMATION OF THE DAY:

WHAT DO I NEED FROM TODAY'S PRACTICE?

MY INTENTION IS:

AFTER YOGA

TODAY'S PRACTICE INCLUDED:

- ☐ yoga poses (*asana*)
- ☐ breathwork (*pranayama*)
- ☐ meditation (*dhyana*)
- ☐ chanting mantra
- ☐ other: ________

3 WORDS THAT CAPTURE HOW MY PRACTICE WENT:

HOW DID THIS PRACTICE AFFECT MY ENERGY LEVELS?

OTHER THOUGHTS:

BEFORE YOGA

DATE ___/___/___

AFFIRMATION OF THE DAY:

WHAT DO I NEED FROM TODAY'S PRACTICE?

MY INTENTION IS:

AFTER YOGA

TODAY'S PRACTICE INCLUDED:

- ☐ yoga poses (*asana*)
- ☐ breathwork (*pranayama*)
- ☐ meditation (*dhyana*)
- ☐ chanting mantra
- ☐ other: ________

3 WORDS THAT CAPTURE HOW MY PRACTICE WENT:

HOW DOES YOGA CONNECT ME WITH MY PURPOSE?

OTHER THOUGHTS:

BEFORE YOGA

DATE ___/___/___

AFFIRMATION OF THE DAY:

WHAT DO I NEED FROM TODAY'S PRACTICE?

MY INTENTION IS:

AFTER YOGA

TODAY'S PRACTICE INCLUDED:

- ☐ yoga poses (*asana*)
- ☐ breathwork (*pranayama*)
- ☐ meditation (*dhyana*)
- ☐ chanting mantra
- ☐ other: __________

3 WORDS THAT CAPTURE HOW MY PRACTICE WENT:

WHAT STOOD OUT MOST ABOUT TODAY'S PRACTICE?

OTHER THOUGHTS:

BEFORE YOGA

DATE ___/___/___

AFFIRMATION OF THE DAY:

WHAT DO I NEED FROM TODAY'S PRACTICE?

MY INTENTION IS:

AFTER YOGA

TODAY'S PRACTICE INCLUDED:

- ☐ yoga poses (*asana*)
- ☐ breathwork (*pranayama*)
- ☐ meditation (*dhyana*)
- ☐ chanting mantra
- ☐ other: ______

3 WORDS THAT CAPTURE HOW MY PRACTICE WENT:

WHAT AM I MOST PROUD OF?

OTHER THOUGHTS:

BEFORE YOGA

DATE ___/___/___

AFFIRMATION OF THE DAY:

WHAT DO I NEED FROM TODAY'S PRACTICE?

MY INTENTION IS:

AFTER YOGA

TODAY'S PRACTICE INCLUDED:

- ☐ yoga poses (*asana*)
- ☐ breathwork (*pranayama*)
- ☐ meditation (*dhyana*)
- ☐ chanting mantra
- ☐ other: ___

3 WORDS THAT CAPTURE HOW MY PRACTICE WENT:

WHAT WAS THE HARDEST PART OF TODAY'S PRACTICE?

OTHER THOUGHTS:

BEFORE YOGA

DATE ___/___/___

AFFIRMATION OF THE DAY:

WHAT DO I NEED FROM TODAY'S PRACTICE?

MY INTENTION IS:

AFTER YOGA

TODAY'S PRACTICE INCLUDED:

- ☐ yoga poses (*asana*)
- ☐ breathwork (*pranayama*)
- ☐ meditation (*dhyana*)
- ☐ chanting mantra
- ☐ other: ____________

3 WORDS THAT CAPTURE HOW MY PRACTICE WENT:

WHAT DID I LEARN ABOUT MYSELF?

OTHER THOUGHTS:

BEFORE YOGA

DATE ___/___/___

AFFIRMATION OF THE DAY:

WHAT DO I NEED FROM TODAY'S PRACTICE?

MY INTENTION IS:

AFTER YOGA

TODAY'S PRACTICE INCLUDED:

- ☐ yoga poses (*asana*)
- ☐ breathwork (*pranayama*)
- ☐ meditation (*dhyana*)
- ☐ chanting mantra
- ☐ other: ___________

3 WORDS THAT CAPTURE HOW MY PRACTICE WENT:

HOW CAN I TAKE MY YOGA OFF THE MAT AND INTO THE WORLD?

OTHER THOUGHTS:

BEFORE YOGA

DATE ___/___/___

AFFIRMATION OF THE DAY:

WHAT DO I NEED FROM TODAY'S PRACTICE?

MY INTENTION IS:

AFTER YOGA

TODAY'S PRACTICE INCLUDED:

- ☐ yoga poses (*asana*)
- ☐ breathwork (*pranayama*)
- ☐ meditation (*dhyana*)
- ☐ chanting mantra
- ☐ other: ___

3 WORDS THAT CAPTURE HOW MY PRACTICE WENT:

WHAT DOES YOGA MEAN TO ME?

OTHER THOUGHTS:

BEFORE YOGA

DATE ___/___/___

AFFIRMATION OF THE DAY:

WHAT DO I NEED FROM TODAY'S PRACTICE?

MY INTENTION IS:

AFTER YOGA

TODAY'S PRACTICE INCLUDED:

- ☐ yoga poses (*asana*)
- ☐ breathwork (*pranayama*)
- ☐ meditation (*dhyana*)
- ☐ chanting mantra
- ☐ other: ___

3 WORDS THAT CAPTURE HOW MY PRACTICE WENT:

HOW CONNECTED WAS I TO MY BREATH?

OTHER THOUGHTS:

BEFORE YOGA

DATE ___/___/___

AFFIRMATION OF THE DAY:

WHAT DO I NEED FROM TODAY'S PRACTICE?

MY INTENTION IS:

AFTER YOGA

TODAY'S PRACTICE INCLUDED:

- ☐ yoga poses (*asana*)
- ☐ breathwork (*pranayama*)
- ☐ meditation (*dhyana*)
- ☐ chanting mantra
- ☐ other: ____________

3 WORDS THAT CAPTURE HOW MY PRACTICE WENT:

HOW DO I FEEL ABOUT MY BODY RIGHT NOW?

OTHER THOUGHTS:

BEFORE YOGA

DATE ___/___/___

AFFIRMATION OF THE DAY:

WHAT DO I NEED FROM TODAY'S PRACTICE?

MY INTENTION IS:

AFTER YOGA

TODAY'S PRACTICE INCLUDED:

- ☐ yoga poses (*asana*)
- ☐ breathwork (*pranayama*)
- ☐ meditation (*dhyana*)
- ☐ chanting mantra
- ☐ other: ___

3 WORDS THAT CAPTURE HOW MY PRACTICE WENT:

DID I HONOR MY INTENTION DURING PRACTICE?

OTHER THOUGHTS:

BEFORE YOGA

DATE ___/___/___

AFFIRMATION OF THE DAY:

WHAT DO I NEED FROM TODAY'S PRACTICE?

MY INTENTION IS:

AFTER YOGA

TODAY'S PRACTICE INCLUDED:

- ☐ yoga poses (*asana*)
- ☐ breathwork (*pranayama*)
- ☐ meditation (*dhyana*)
- ☐ chanting mantra
- ☐ other: __________

3 WORDS THAT CAPTURE HOW MY PRACTICE WENT:

WHAT WAS THE MAIN EMOTION FELT DURING PRACTICE?

OTHER THOUGHTS:

BEFORE YOGA

DATE ___/___/___

AFFIRMATION OF THE DAY:

____

WHAT DO I NEED FROM TODAY'S PRACTICE?

____

____

____

MY INTENTION IS:

____

____

AFTER YOGA

TODAY'S PRACTICE INCLUDED:

- ☐ yoga poses (*asana*)
- ☐ breathwork (*pranayama*)
- ☐ meditation (*dhyana*)
- ☐ chanting mantra
- ☐ other: ___________

3 WORDS THAT CAPTURE HOW MY PRACTICE WENT:

____

____

____

HOW DO I REACT WHEN FACED WITH A CHALLENGING POSE OR PRACTICE?

____

____

____

OTHER THOUGHTS:

____

____

____

BEFORE YOGA

DATE ___/___/___

AFFIRMATION OF THE DAY:

WHAT DO I NEED FROM TODAY'S PRACTICE?

MY INTENTION IS:

AFTER YOGA

TODAY'S PRACTICE INCLUDED:

- ☐ yoga poses (*asana*)
- ☐ breathwork (*pranayama*)
- ☐ meditation (*dhyana*)
- ☐ chanting mantra
- ☐ other: ___

3 WORDS THAT CAPTURE HOW MY PRACTICE WENT:

HOW ARE EVENTS IN MY LIFE AFFECTING MY PRACTICE?

OTHER THOUGHTS:

BEFORE YOGA

DATE ___/___/___

AFFIRMATION OF THE DAY:

WHAT DO I NEED FROM TODAY'S PRACTICE?

MY INTENTION IS:

AFTER YOGA

TODAY'S PRACTICE INCLUDED:

- ☐ yoga poses (*asana*)
- ☐ breathwork (*pranayama*)
- ☐ meditation (*dhyana*)
- ☐ chanting mantra
- ☐ other: ______

3 WORDS THAT CAPTURE HOW MY PRACTICE WENT:

HOW DOES MY PRACTICE AFFECT MY DAY-TO-DAY LIFE?

OTHER THOUGHTS:

BEFORE YOGA

DATE ___/___/___

AFFIRMATION OF THE DAY:

WHAT DO I NEED FROM TODAY'S PRACTICE?

MY INTENTION IS:

AFTER YOGA

TODAY'S PRACTICE INCLUDED:

- ☐ yoga poses (*asana*)
- ☐ breathwork (*pranayama*)
- ☐ meditation (*dhyana*)
- ☐ chanting mantra
- ☐ other: ______________

3 WORDS THAT CAPTURE HOW MY PRACTICE WENT:

HOW CAN I USE THIS PRACTICE FOR SPIRITUAL GROWTH?

OTHER THOUGHTS:

BEFORE YOGA

DATE ___/___/___

AFFIRMATION OF THE DAY:

WHAT DO I NEED FROM TODAY'S PRACTICE?

MY INTENTION IS:

AFTER YOGA

TODAY'S PRACTICE INCLUDED:

- ☐ yoga poses (*asana*)
- ☐ breathwork (*pranayama*)
- ☐ meditation (*dhyana*)
- ☐ chanting mantra
- ☐ other: __________

3 WORDS THAT CAPTURE HOW MY PRACTICE WENT:

HOW EASY OR DIFFICULT WAS IT FOR ME TO STAY FOCUSED?

OTHER THOUGHTS:

BEFORE YOGA

DATE ___/___/___

AFFIRMATION OF THE DAY:

WHAT DO I NEED FROM TODAY'S PRACTICE?

MY INTENTION IS:

AFTER YOGA

TODAY'S PRACTICE INCLUDED:

- ☐ yoga poses (*asana*)
- ☐ breathwork (*pranayama*)
- ☐ meditation (*dhyana*)
- ☐ chanting mantra
- ☐ other: ___

3 WORDS THAT CAPTURE HOW MY PRACTICE WENT:

WHAT HELPS ME STAY IN THE PRESENT MOMENT?

OTHER THOUGHTS:

BEFORE YOGA

DATE ___/___/___

AFFIRMATION OF THE DAY:

WHAT DO I NEED FROM TODAY'S PRACTICE?

MY INTENTION IS:

AFTER YOGA

TODAY'S PRACTICE INCLUDED:

- ☐ yoga poses (*asana*)
- ☐ breathwork (*pranayama*)
- ☐ meditation (*dhyana*)
- ☐ chanting mantra
- ☐ other: ___

3 WORDS THAT CAPTURE HOW MY PRACTICE WENT:

WHICH TEACHERS DO I FIND MOST INSPIRING AND WHY?

OTHER THOUGHTS:

BEFORE YOGA

DATE ___/___/___

AFFIRMATION OF THE DAY:

WHAT DO I NEED FROM TODAY'S PRACTICE?

MY INTENTION IS:

AFTER YOGA

TODAY'S PRACTICE INCLUDED:

- ☐ yoga poses (*asana*)
- ☐ breathwork (*pranayama*)
- ☐ meditation (*dhyana*)
- ☐ chanting mantra
- ☐ other: ___

3 WORDS THAT CAPTURE HOW MY PRACTICE WENT:

IF I COULD CHANGE ANYTHING FROM TODAY'S PRACTICE, WHAT WOULD IT BE?

OTHER THOUGHTS:

BEFORE YOGA

DATE ___/___/___

AFFIRMATION OF THE DAY:

WHAT DO I NEED FROM TODAY'S PRACTICE?

MY INTENTION IS:

AFTER YOGA

TODAY'S PRACTICE INCLUDED:

- ☐ yoga poses (*asana*)
- ☐ breathwork (*pranayama*)
- ☐ meditation (*dhyana*)
- ☐ chanting mantra
- ☐ other: ___

3 WORDS THAT CAPTURE HOW MY PRACTICE WENT:

DO I TEND TO PUSH TOO HARD OR HOLD BACK?

OTHER THOUGHTS:

BEFORE YOGA

DATE ___/___/___

AFFIRMATION OF THE DAY:

WHAT DO I NEED FROM TODAY'S PRACTICE?

MY INTENTION IS:

AFTER YOGA

TODAY'S PRACTICE INCLUDED:

- ☐ yoga poses (*asana*)
- ☐ breathwork (*pranayama*)
- ☐ meditation (*dhyana*)
- ☐ chanting mantra
- ☐ other: __________

3 WORDS THAT CAPTURE HOW MY PRACTICE WENT:

WHAT MOTIVATES ME TO KEEP PRACTICING EVERY DAY?

OTHER THOUGHTS:

BEFORE YOGA

DATE ___/___/___

AFFIRMATION OF THE DAY:

WHAT DO I NEED FROM TODAY'S PRACTICE?

MY INTENTION IS:

AFTER YOGA

TODAY'S PRACTICE INCLUDED:

- ☐ yoga poses (*asana*)
- ☐ breathwork (*pranayama*)
- ☐ meditation (*dhyana*)
- ☐ chanting mantra
- ☐ other: ___

3 WORDS THAT CAPTURE HOW MY PRACTICE WENT:

HOW HAS MY RELATIONSHIP WITH YOGA CHANGED WITH TIME?

OTHER THOUGHTS:

BEFORE YOGA

DATE ___/___/___

AFFIRMATION OF THE DAY:

WHAT DO I NEED FROM TODAY'S PRACTICE?

MY INTENTION IS:

AFTER YOGA

TODAY'S PRACTICE INCLUDED:

- ☐ yoga poses (*asana*)
- ☐ breathwork (*pranayama*)
- ☐ meditation (*dhyana*)
- ☐ chanting mantra
- ☐ other: ______________

3 WORDS THAT CAPTURE HOW MY PRACTICE WENT:

WHAT DO I NEED MORE OF IN MY PRACTICE?

OTHER THOUGHTS:

BEFORE YOGA

DATE ___/___/___

AFFIRMATION OF THE DAY:

WHAT DO I NEED FROM TODAY'S PRACTICE?

MY INTENTION IS:

AFTER YOGA

TODAY'S PRACTICE INCLUDED:

- ☐ yoga poses (*asana*)
- ☐ breathwork (*pranayama*)
- ☐ meditation (*dhyana*)
- ☐ chanting mantra
- ☐ other: ___

3 WORDS THAT CAPTURE HOW MY PRACTICE WENT:

WHAT DO I WANT TO WORK ON NEXT TIME?

OTHER THOUGHTS:

BEFORE YOGA

DATE ___/___/___

AFFIRMATION OF THE DAY:

WHAT DO I NEED FROM TODAY'S PRACTICE?

MY INTENTION IS:

AFTER YOGA

TODAY'S PRACTICE INCLUDED:

- ☐ yoga poses (*asana*)
- ☐ breathwork (*pranayama*)
- ☐ meditation (*dhyana*)
- ☐ chanting mantra
- ☐ other: ___________

3 WORDS THAT CAPTURE HOW MY PRACTICE WENT:

AM I NEGLECTING AN IMPORTANT ASPECT OF MY YOGA PRACTICE?

OTHER THOUGHTS:

BEFORE YOGA

DATE ___/___/___

AFFIRMATION OF THE DAY:

____

WHAT DO I NEED FROM TODAY'S PRACTICE?

____

____

____

MY INTENTION IS:

____

____

AFTER YOGA

TODAY'S PRACTICE INCLUDED:

- ☐ yoga poses (*asana*)
- ☐ breathwork (*pranayama*)
- ☐ meditation (*dhyana*)
- ☐ chanting mantra
- ☐ other: ______________

3 WORDS THAT CAPTURE HOW MY PRACTICE WENT:

____

____

____

DOES MY INTERNAL DIALOGUE TEND TO BE POSITIVE OR NEGATIVE?

____

____

____

OTHER THOUGHTS:

____

____

____

BEFORE YOGA

DATE ___/___/___

AFFIRMATION OF THE DAY:

WHAT DO I NEED FROM TODAY'S PRACTICE?

MY INTENTION IS:

AFTER YOGA

TODAY'S PRACTICE INCLUDED:

- ☐ yoga poses (*asana*)
- ☐ breathwork (*pranayama*)
- ☐ meditation (*dhyana*)
- ☐ chanting mantra
- ☐ other: __________

3 WORDS THAT CAPTURE HOW MY PRACTICE WENT:

WHAT AM I MOST GRATEFUL FOR RIGHT NOW?

OTHER THOUGHTS:

BEFORE YOGA

DATE ___/___/___

AFFIRMATION OF THE DAY:

WHAT DO I NEED FROM TODAY'S PRACTICE?

MY INTENTION IS:

AFTER YOGA

TODAY'S PRACTICE INCLUDED:

- ☐ yoga poses (*asana*)
- ☐ breathwork (*pranayama*)
- ☐ meditation (*dhyana*)
- ☐ chanting mantra
- ☐ other: ___

3 WORDS THAT CAPTURE HOW MY PRACTICE WENT:

WHAT IS SOMETHING I NEED TO STUDY DEEPER?

OTHER THOUGHTS:

BEFORE YOGA

DATE ___/___/___

AFFIRMATION OF THE DAY:

WHAT DO I NEED FROM TODAY'S PRACTICE?

MY INTENTION IS:

AFTER YOGA

TODAY'S PRACTICE INCLUDED:

- ☐ yoga poses (*asana*)
- ☐ breathwork (*pranayama*)
- ☐ meditation (*dhyana*)
- ☐ chanting mantra
- ☐ other: ___________

3 WORDS THAT CAPTURE HOW MY PRACTICE WENT:

HOW DOES YOGA AFFECT MY EMOTIONAL HEALTH?

OTHER THOUGHTS:

BEFORE YOGA

DATE ___/___/___

AFFIRMATION OF THE DAY:

WHAT DO I NEED FROM TODAY'S PRACTICE?

MY INTENTION IS:

AFTER YOGA

TODAY'S PRACTICE INCLUDED:

- ☐ yoga poses (*asana*)
- ☐ breathwork (*pranayama*)
- ☐ meditation (*dhyana*)
- ☐ chanting mantra
- ☐ other: ___________

3 WORDS THAT CAPTURE HOW MY PRACTICE WENT:

HOW DID THIS PRACTICE AFFECT MY ENERGY LEVELS?

OTHER THOUGHTS:

BEFORE YOGA

DATE ___/___/___

AFFIRMATION OF THE DAY:

WHAT DO I NEED FROM TODAY'S PRACTICE?

MY INTENTION IS:

AFTER YOGA

TODAY'S PRACTICE INCLUDED:

- ☐ yoga poses (*asana*)
- ☐ breathwork (*pranayama*)
- ☐ meditation (*dhyana*)
- ☐ chanting mantra
- ☐ other: ___

3 WORDS THAT CAPTURE HOW MY PRACTICE WENT:

HOW DOES YOGA CONNECT ME WITH MY PURPOSE?

OTHER THOUGHTS:

BEFORE YOGA

DATE ___/___/___

AFFIRMATION OF THE DAY:

WHAT DO I NEED FROM TODAY'S PRACTICE?

MY INTENTION IS:

AFTER YOGA

TODAY'S PRACTICE INCLUDED:

- ☐ yoga poses (*asana*)
- ☐ breathwork (*pranayama*)
- ☐ meditation (*dhyana*)
- ☐ chanting mantra
- ☐ other: ___

3 WORDS THAT CAPTURE HOW MY PRACTICE WENT:

WHAT STOOD OUT MOST ABOUT TODAY'S PRACTICE?

OTHER THOUGHTS:

BEFORE YOGA

DATE ___/___/___

AFFIRMATION OF THE DAY:

WHAT DO I NEED FROM TODAY'S PRACTICE?

MY INTENTION IS:

AFTER YOGA

TODAY'S PRACTICE INCLUDED:

- ☐ yoga poses (*asana*)
- ☐ breathwork (*pranayama*)
- ☐ meditation (*dhyana*)
- ☐ chanting mantra
- ☐ other: ___

3 WORDS THAT CAPTURE HOW MY PRACTICE WENT:

WHAT AM I MOST PROUD OF?

OTHER THOUGHTS:

BEFORE YOGA

DATE ___/___/___

AFFIRMATION OF THE DAY:

WHAT DO I NEED FROM TODAY'S PRACTICE?

MY INTENTION IS:

AFTER YOGA

TODAY'S PRACTICE INCLUDED:

- ☐ yoga poses (*asana*)
- ☐ breathwork (*pranayama*)
- ☐ meditation (*dhyana*)
- ☐ chanting mantra
- ☐ other: __________

3 WORDS THAT CAPTURE HOW MY PRACTICE WENT:

WHAT WAS THE HARDEST PART OF TODAY'S PRACTICE?

OTHER THOUGHTS: